What You Need to Know about Autism

What You Need to Know about Autism

Christopher M. Cumo

Inside Diseases and Disorders

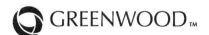 GREENWOOD™

An Imprint of ABC-CLIO, LLC
Santa Barbara, California • Denver, Colorado

Library of Congress Cataloging-in-Publication Data
Names: Cumo, Christopher, author.
Title: What you need to know about autism / Christopher M. Cumo.
Description: Santa Barbara, California : Greenwood, [2019] | Series: Inside
    diseases and disorders | Includes bibliographical references and index. |
Identifiers: LCCN 2018031659 (print) | LCCN 2018035088 (ebook) |
    ISBN 9781440862939 (eBook) | ISBN 9781440862922 (hard copy : alk. paper)
Subjects: LCSH: Autism. | Autism—Treatment. | Autistic people—Family
    relationships. | Autism—Case studies.
Classification: LCC RC553.A88 (ebook) | LCC RC553.A88 C86 2019 (print) | DDC
    616.85/882—dc23
LC record available at https://lccn.loc.gov/2018031659

ISBN: 978-1-4408-6292-2 (print)
        978-1-4408-6293-9 (ebook)

23 22 21 20 19   1 2 3 4 5

This book is also available as an eBook.

Greenwood
An Imprint of ABC-CLIO, LLC

ABC-CLIO, LLC
130 Cremona Drive, P.O. Box 1911
Santa Barbara, California 93116-1911
www.abc-clio.com

This book is printed on acid-free paper ∞

Manufactured in the United States of America

Contents

Series Foreword

Disease is as old as humanity itself, and it has been the leading cause of death and disability throughout history. From the Black Death in the Middle Ages to smallpox outbreaks among Native Americans to the modern-day epidemics of diabetes and heart disease, humans have lived with—and died from—all manner of ailments, whether caused by infectious agents, environmental and lifestyle factors, or genetic abnormalities. The field of medicine has been driven forward by our desire to combat and prevent disease and to improve the lives of those living with debilitating disorders. And while we have made great strides forward, particularly in the last 100 years, it is doubtful that mankind will ever be completely free of the burden of disease.

Greenwood's Inside Diseases and Disorders series examines some of the key diseases and disorders, both physical and psychological, affecting the world today. Some (such as diabetes, cardiovascular disease, and ADHD) have been selected because of their prominence within modern America. Others (such as Ebola, celiac disease, and autism) have been chosen because they are often discussed in the media and, in some cases, are controversial or the subject of scientific or cultural debate.

Because this series covers so many different diseases and disorders, we have striven to create uniformity across all books. To maximize clarity and consistency, each book in the series follows the same format. Each begins with a collection of 10 frequently asked questions about the disease or disorder, followed by clear, concise answers. Chapter 1 provides a general introduction to the disease or disorder, including statistical information such as prevalence rates and demographic trends. The history of the disease or disorder, including how our understanding of it has evolved over time, is addressed in chapter 2. Chapter 3 examines causes and risk factors, whether genetic, microbial, or environmental, while chapter 4 discusses signs and symptoms. Chapter 5 covers the issues of diagnosis (and misdiagnosis), treatment, and management (whether with drugs, medical procedures, or lifestyle changes). How such treatment, or the lack thereof, affects a patient's long-term prognosis, as well as the risk of complications, are the subject of chapter 6. Chapter 7 explores the disease or disorder's effects on the friends and family of a patient—a dimension often over-looked in discussions of physical and psychological ailments. Chapter 8 discusses prevention strategies, while chapter 9 explores key issues or con-troversies, whether medical or sociocultural. Finally, chapter 10 profiles cutting-edge research and speculates on how things might change in the next few decades.

Each volume also features five fictional case studies to illustrate differ-ent aspects of the book's subject matter, highlighting key concepts and themes that have been explored throughout the text. The reader will also find a glossary of terms and a collection of print and electronic resources for additional information and further study.

As a final caveat, please be aware that the information presented in these books is no substitute for consultation with a licensed health care professional. These books do not claim to provide medical advice or guidance.

Acknowledgments

My association with ABC-CLIO goes back many years. I am fortunate to have the confidence and support of its staff. Among them, Health and Wellness senior acquisitions editor Maxine Taylor deserves my gratitude for giving me the opportunity to write this book, which has benefitted from her guidance in the journey from concept to product. Her hard work helped realize this book.

My local library, the Stark County District Library in Canton, Ohio, also merits mention. Its librarians helped me locate suitable resources. Their advice led me to consult books, articles, websites, and other items that might have escaped my notice. Additionally, the library lets patrons borrow books and other media from Ohio's public, college, and university libraries, allowing me access to materials that would otherwise have been beyond my reach. Although not a research institution, the Stark County District Library functions enough like one for my purposes.

The greatest thanks, love, devotion, affection, and admiration are due my wife, Dietra, and my daughters Francesca and Allie. They are the most important people in my life, and their support has helped me through difficulties. Their example encourages me to be a better person. I can never hope to express all they mean to me.

Introduction

This book's impetus came from the recognition that autism, better labeled autism spectrum disorder (ASD), is a worldwide story with many actors, opinions, attitudes, perspectives, and perceptions. As is true of anything vital and dynamic, ASD's saga must be told and retold as new knowledge and hypotheses emerge.

My desire to write *What You Need to Know about Autism* stems partly from the belief that a compelling story never grows old. Fresh perspectives abound, challenging writers, scientists, and medical practitioners to share what they have learned. Most of these accounts have their genesis in the reflections of clinicians and others who observe patients with ASD and comb the literature for insights into the condition. Such reflections are secondhand in the sense that the writer does not live with ASD. This statement is not a criticism because these authors may be more dispassionate than those who struggle against ASD.

I too have tried to be dispassionate, even antiseptic, but I have not attempted to write about ASD from a distance. My experiences as a 54-year-old autistic man convince me that ASD shapes in some measure what it means to be human, at least for a sizable minority of us. Natural selection endowed us with a large brain to crown an intricate central nervous system (CNS). But as with anything complex—a luxury automobile for example—much can go wrong and the consequences can be disastrous and expensive. Being a neurological condition, ASD illustrates the perils of a CNS whose functioning and fine tuning are impaired to greater or lesser extent.

The range of ASD's signs and symptoms compel the realization that it is a spectrum rather than a rigid phenomenon. The bewildering array of signs and symptoms challenges even the best diagnostician. Accordingly, diagnosis is as much art as science and medicine. Although, as this book and other literature emphasize, most cases are identified by the second or third year of life, some people with ASD evade detection for decades.

Suffering from depression and anxiety, I went through a long list of general practitioners, psychiatrists, hospitals, and medicines. The professionals thought, as I did, that I displayed classic traits of a clinically depressed and anxious person. The only question was whether I was bipolar or unipolar. Such labels meant nothing to me. I just wanted relief. In my forties I visited a young psychiatrist fresh out of his residency. Within a few minutes of our first meeting he diagnosed me with Asperger's syndrome, which was then a stand-alone condition. Asperger's syndrome, now integrated into ASD, makes me what one psychologist termed a "high-functioning autistic."

Such language, again, is an exercise in labeling. From this perspective, names are unimportant. Yet at a deeper level, an ASD diagnosis gave me a path to pursue. Mindful of others' conviction that I had no insight into myself, I began reading about ASD in hopes of remedying this deficiency. After all, Greek philosopher Plato reminds us in the *Apology* of the need for self-knowledge. Such knowledge appears to be a foundation for learning about the world outside ourselves. English philosopher Francis Bacon believed that knowledge empowers people. But power comes from application. An esoteric accounting of the world or something in it accomplishes nothing. Given this reality, I wanted to learn about ASD as prelude to improving my life.

But I could not stop at myself because humans are social animals. Although craving solitude and introspection, I live amid others whose opinions about me matter despite my wish otherwise. They have always vexed me, perhaps because I have trouble decoding nonverbal cues. From childhood, whatever others have said and done has surprised and sometimes shocked me because of my inability to fathom their intentions.

Such intentions can be sinister. One problem with having ASD or another serious condition is people's tendency to undervalue disabled persons. Even after I had earned a PhD and published a number of books and articles, my father advised me to seek work at McDonald's. He never wavered from this conviction or explained his rationale, but I suspect he doubted my ability to do anything else.

Unkind evaluations dishearten their recipient. Although I never worked at McDonald's, I spent nearly 40 years cutting grass. Evidently my father's dour assessment is pervasive enough to prompt potential employers to discard my CV. No one has hired me to do another job even with an education and publications. In cutting grass until osteoarthritis and bone spurs hobbled me, I legitimized my doubters.

These experiences have taught me that ASD studies, if such language is permissible, needs autistic authors to saturate the market with success stories, an approach suitable for people with other disabilities. The effort to give voice to marginalized people should put ASD literature on par with scholarship about women, minorities, and other disadvantaged groups. Books and articles along these lines might even counteract the tendency to devalue those of us with disabilities.

This book thus treats ASD as more than a disability or set of implacable limits. As do other disabled people, many people with ASD surmount difficulties en route to successful careers and independent lives. True, the proportion of unemployed and underemployed people with ASD is alarming, but statistics are not destiny. No autistic person is content to be relegated to the sidelines while others enjoy life. Individuals with ASD aim to participate fully in life's adventures.

What You Need to Know about Autism celebrates autistic people as it informs the reader about their experiences. The book educates high school students and undergraduates in hopes that an informed citizenry is best suited to construct policies that maximize the potential of everyone, including those with ASD and other disabled people. This book hopes to instill compassion so that readers will not judge harshly. Understanding and compassion need not be scarce. They typify those who reap education's true benefits.

Essential Questions

1. ARE AUTISM AND AUTISM SPECTRUM DISORDER (ASD) DIFFERENT CONDITIONS?

Autism and ASD are labels for a neurological condition that affects the body, intellect, behavior, communication, and sociability. Between 1911 and 2012 the term "autism" described this malady. In 2013 the fifth edition of the *Diagnostic Statistical Manual of Mental Disorders* replaced "autism" with "autism spectrum disorder" to emphasize that the signs and symptoms lie on a continuum. Rather than being a discrete phenomenon, ASD is best thought of as a spectrum of problems. Chapter 1's section "Toward a Definition of Autism" defines the condition in detail. The rest of the chapter pinpoints its effects on the body. Chapter 2's section "Movement toward Recognition That ASD Is a Spectrum of Disorders" details the transition in thinking that led to "ASD" as the current label for autism.

2. WHY DOES ASD VARY MARKEDLY IN SEVERITY FROM PERSON TO PERSON?

Research suggests that genetics play a prominent role in ASD. A large number of genes appear to be involved. The fewer the number of harmful genes, the greater is the likelihood that signs and symptoms will be mild. The addition of more harmful genes increases the probability that signs and symptoms will grow in severity. Because such a large number of genes are at issue, people inherit vastly different combinations and amounts of them, producing a range of severities. Chapter 3's section "Genetics" describes the role of genes in ASD. All of Chapter 4, especially the section "Signs and Symptoms on the Spectrum" describes variability in severity.

3. WHAT CAUSES ASD?

ASD results from the interaction of genetic and environmental factors, detailed in Chapter 3.

4. WHAT IS THE PROGNOSIS FOR SOMEONE WITH ASD?

Prognosis depends on the severity of signs and symptoms and the efficacy of treatment and management. People with ASD with the worst symptoms, the poor, and minorities tend to have dour prognoses. Chapter 5's section "Treatment and Management" details the best strategies to minimize signs and symptoms over short and long terms. Chapter 9's sections "The Economy" and "Race" document the reality that the poor and minorities face barriers to treatment. Chapter 9's section "Longevity" documents the fact that people with ASD tend to die sooner than neurotypical persons.

5. CAN ASD BE PREVENTED?

Given the current state of science and medicine, ASD cannot be prevented. Chapter 8 details and evaluates efforts to prevent ASD.

6. WHY DO MORE BOYS THAN GIRLS SUFFER FROM ASD?

Boys are roughly five times more likely than girls to have ASD because genes on the X chromosome, a sex chromosome, appear to contribute to ASD's onset and severity. Boys and girls have different couplings of sex chromosomes, leading to this disparity. Chapter 1's section "ASD in Children and Adults" explains how the pairing of genes on the X chromosome contributes to ASD.

7. WHAT ARE ASD'S PRINCIPAL SIGNS AND SYMPTOMS?

Signs and symptoms may be numerous and often vary in severity. Physical, intellectual, communication, sensory, behavioral, and social signs and symptoms mark someone as having ASD. Chapter 4 details prominent signs and symptoms.

8. WHAT TREATMENTS WORK BEST AGAINST ASD?

ASD's marked variations among people complicate any attempt to generalize about the efficacy of one treatment versus another. Treatments fall into the categories of pharmacology, diet, and behavior. To date, dietary modifications have not been shown to be effective in clinical trials despite the availability of anecdotes that describe success. Neither pharmacological nor behavioral therapies can boast great success. The current status of these therapies leads to the conclusion that scientists and medical practitioners need to understand ASD in greater detail in hopes of tailoring the best treatment to each individual. A one-size-fits-all model is unlikely to succeed. Because genes play a role in ASD, gene therapy appears to be the ultimate but as yet unrealized treatment for the condition. Chapter 5's section "Treatment and Management" details and evaluates current treatments.

9. DO VACCINES CAUSE ASD?

Despite the claims of a 1998 publication, vaccines do not cause ASD. Chapter 9 details the controversy about vaccines in its section "Vaccination."

10. HOW CAN FAMILY AND FRIENDS HELP LOVED ONES WITH ASD?

Family and friends play an important role in helping loved ones with ASD cope with life's demands. ASD places social, logistical, and financial burdens on families. Stress and fatigue can strain marriages, demanding that parents rely on grandparents and other caregivers to lighten their load. Research suggests that family members and friends who join support groups are often better able to help their loved ones. The camaraderie of such groups helps alleviate the isolation that too often mars quality of life for family and friends. Chapter 7 details ASD's effects on family and friends and ways these people can help their loved ones with ASD.

1

What Is Autism?

Cases of autism appear to be on the rise, and the condition has become a hot topic for discussion in both medical and media circles. Despite this current interest in autism, the condition is not new—medical professionals have been observing and trying to understand the signs and symptoms of autism for hundreds of years. Autism sinks deep roots into the past, as is evident in the word "autism," which derives from the Greek word *autos*, itself an ancient word that might be translated as "the self," in recognition of the fact that an autistic person often lacks social skills and so becomes an isolated self. This chapter explores what autism is, its defining characteristics, and its prevalence. It is important to remember, however, that autism occurs along a spectrum and can manifest in very different ways from person to person.

TOWARD A DEFINITION OF AUTISM

Mental health practitioners do not define autism as a single disease, condition, ailment, affliction, or malady but rather as many related disorders, known collectively as autism spectrum disorder (ASD), sometimes rendered autism spectrum disorders. The attributes that unite these disorders under a single umbrella include developmental and neurological deficits because, at its core, ASD is a neurological condition.

The National Institute of Mental Health characterizes autism as a social disorder, which is appropriate given the social deficits of ASD. In general, humans are social beings by nature. They tend to gravitate towards one another, exchanging information, building networks, and building cities and civilizations along the way. But these momentous connections elude autistic people, who have difficulty with social interactions. They may have trouble, for example, holding a conversation or making eye contact with other people. Other traits may include a tendency to repeat behaviors to the point of repeating actions that harm themselves, like repeatedly banging their head against a wall. The tendency toward self-harm is known as self-injurious behaviors. Autistic people may have a narrow set of interests or activities in comparison with many nonautistic people. Although the onset of autism may vary, the typical person displays signs and symptoms early, usually before or by age two.

The classification of autism as a range of disorders has shaped the way people think about it. In the past mental health practitioners were inclined to place in separate categories disorders that now fall under the umbrella of ASD. In this context it is important to note that what was formerly known as Asperger's syndrome, as well as other similar disorders, were grouped into the larger category of ASD in the 2013 *Diagnostic and Statistical Manual of Mental Disorders*, the *DSM-5*. For this reason, it seems more accurate to use the label "ASD" rather than the term "autism" in referring to the range of signs and symptoms that characterizes it.

ASD'S EFFECTS ON THE BODY

Mental health practitioners and researchers are learning more about ASD every day. At this point it seems safe to conclude that ASD affects the body in many ways. Attention has focused on the central nervous system (CNS) because ASD is a neurological condition. The CNS includes all the nerve tissues that regulate the body's activities. In humans and many other animals, the CNS is the brain and spinal cord. The brain is made up of cells known as neurons. Neurons carry messages in the form of chemicals from the brain to other parts of the body. These chemicals travel from one neuron to another by crossing gaps known as synapses. These neurons and synapses play a crucial role in helping scientists and doctors understand ASD, incomplete though this understanding may be.

The brain has a very large number of synapses during early stages in human development. This number appears to diminish during development, although the total number of synapses in a fully developed brain remains large by any accounting. The rate of diminution, especially in adolescence, reveals much about ASD. Research suggests that people with

ASD have more synapses than people without ASD. That is, autistic people seem to have brains that remain at a stage of development before the consolidation of synapses.

It may help to think of the brain and its neurons as a system of connected wires that carry electricity. The analogy is apt because neurons carry electrochemical charges. The wires must conduct this electricity in an orderly way for the system to work well. The neurons of the brain of a person with ASD, however, appear to misfire or to fire inefficiently to some degree, impairing the normal functioning of the brain. These misfirings appear to occur in the regions of the brain known as the corpus callosum, the amygdala, and the cerebellum. These areas perform important functions. The corpus callosum may be envisioned as a bundle of fibers that connects the two hemispheres of the brain. Consequently it facilitates communication between the two halves. The amygdala, deep within the brain's temporal lobes, is the center of emotions. Fear, aggression, and pleasure all seem to originate here. At the back of the skull, the cerebellum coordinates the timing, sequence, and rate of muscle contractions.

Related to the CNS is the neuroendocrine system, which ASD may also harm. The neuroendocrine system includes a complex group of organs, among them the pineal gland, the pituitary gland, the pancreas, the ovaries in women or the testes in men, the thyroid gland, the parathyroid gland, the hypothalamus, and the adrenal glands. Glands produce chemicals known as hormones that regulate certain areas and processes in the body. In the neuroendocrine system, hormones regulate appetite, metabolism, reproduction, osmolarity (the concentration of chemicals in the liquid inside a cell), and blood pressure. ASD may harm the neuroendocrine system in several ways. Prominent among these problems is the over or under stimulation of the body's glands, causing excess or shortage of a hormone or hormones. For example, children tend to experience an increase in the (not anabolic) steroid hormone known as cortisol in the morning, but ASD children often do not experience this change. Because cortisol readies the body for activity it is typically high in the morning to give the body a jolt of energy.

ASD may also afflict the immune system. The immune system is a group of cells that patrol the body to guard against infection. When these cells detect the presence of a foreign particle, like a bacterium, fungus, or virus, they attack it in hopes of eliminating the invader. In autistic people, the immune system does not always work optimally. In such cases, the immune system may mistake other parts of the body for foreign invaders and attack them instead. For example, in autistic people the immune system may attack the brain, causing the brain to swell as a result. The immune system is also important because it helps the brain develop early in life. Because of the immune system's role in development, the brain may not mature

normally in autistic people. ASD appears to lessen the presence of chemicals in the brain that regulate the number and kind of immune cells in the
brain. More research is necessary to understand the interactions between
the immune system and autism may also harm the gastrointestinal system. The gastrointestinal system, also known as the digestive system or
the gastrointestinal tract, comprises several parts of the body: the buccal
cavity, the pharynx, the esophagus, the stomach, and the duodenum. These
organs work together to convert food into the energy a living organism
needs to function. In autistic people, gastrointestinal discomfort may be
frequent and among their most common complaints. Problems include
constipation, diarrhea, or inflammation or irritation of the bowel. The
Centers for Disease Control and Prevention (CDC) in Atlanta, Georgia,
estimates that autistic children are as much as 3.5 times more likely to suffer from diarrhea or constipation than are children without ASD. These
problems may persist because some autistic children cannot verbalize the
source of their distress.

The musculoskeletal system may not be robust in autistic persons.
Movement is impossible without muscles. So elemental is this fact that we
seldom think twice about it as we use muscles and tendons in the hand,
forearm and upper arm to grasp a cup of coffee and raise it to the mouth.
Such action is conscious and willful, even though no thought is given to it.
The reader should not forget, however, that muscles perform a variety of
essential operations, like breathing and movement, on their own and without volition. In sum, the proper functioning of muscles is essential to carrying on life's activities.

Yet the autistic person may be at a disadvantage in this regard. His or
her muscles may be weak and susceptible to fatigue. In a more general
sense, autistic people may suffer from dyspraxia, which is difficulty in the
coordination of muscle movements. This difficulty is rooted in both muscles and brain because the brain coordinates muscle movements. Such
coordination may require a high order of functioning absent in an autistic
person. The result is akin to perpetual clumsiness. Such a deficit may be
difficult to pinpoint because children tend to be clumsy in a variety of situations so that the phenomenon is not unique to autistic children. In the
autistic child, however, the range of clumsiness may include difficulties
balancing, sitting erect, walking, running, grasping an object, sitting down
or rising from a seated position, or starting or stopping an action.

Dyspraxia may also be evident in an autistic person's repetitive actions
that result from his or her frustration with an inability to move in precise
ways, or to articulate words clearly because of difficulties coordinating the
muscles. An intriguing aspect of dyspraxia is the fact that some autistic
people do not display a dominant hand. It may be that such a person cannot coordinate the movement of muscles so that he or she, for example,

would favor the right hand in holding a pencil or pen. Dyspraxia may be particularly troubling because an autistic person, due to poor coordination, may have difficulty carrying out routine tasks as instructed, leading the instructor to conclude, erroneously, that the person with ASD lacks the intelligence to follow directions.

These effects on muscles may weaken the bones. The mechanism at work is not entirely understood. The autistic person, having trouble coordinating muscle activity, may exercise little. It is well studied that regular exercise benefits the bones. Alternatively, he or she, self-conscious of poor coordination, may spend little time outdoors, resulting in insufficient production of vitamin D from sunlight. In either case, bones lose density as a result, causing fractures or osteoporosis at a comparatively young age. To compound matters, autistic people may consume fewer foods rich in vitamin D and calcium than do people without ASD, an inadequately understood phenomenon. Bones require both vitamin D and the mineral calcium (a metal on the Periodic Table) for optimal growth, durability, and function.

ASD AFFECTS MANY PEOPLE AROUND THE WORLD

A surge in the number of cases of ASD since the early twenty-first century makes important the attempt to gauge its magnitude. Research on the number of cases of ASD has been intensive in many areas of the world, including the United States, while being deficient in others. Even in the United States, imprecision remains because research reveals a range of estimates rather than a single number. For example, the CDC has reported that 1 in 68 American children have ASD whereas a federal health survey has put the ratio at 1 in 45. Conversion of these ratios into an estimate of the number of autistic Americans requires two steps. First it is necessary to estimate the number of autistic adults in the United States. This task is not impossible because ASD does not now have a cure. Because ASD has no cure, every autistic child should grow into an autistic adult, if it is permissible to ignore childhood mortality. Of course, the severity of signs and symptoms may change during the transition from childhood to adulthood, but these changes do not mean that ASD disappears. In other words, the ratio of autistic adults in the United States should be roughly the same as the ratio of autistic children. With a population of roughly 325 million citizens, the United States should have somewhere between 4.8 and 7.2 million autistic people.

Canada and Mexico also are part of North America. As in the United States, the ratio of autistic Canadians varies, with the latest estimate coming in at 1 in 68 people. With a population of roughly 36 million people,

Canada has approximately 530,000 autistic citizens. Mexico yields a smaller number than either the United States or Canada. With an estimated 1 in 115 Mexicans with ASD and a population at roughly 128 million, Mexico has approximately 1.1 million autistic people.

The situation in South America is difficult to disentangle because estimates vary by country. In fact, few South American countries have been surveyed, leading to spotty data. For example, various agencies have estimated the percentage of ASD cases in Ecuador to be roughly 0.11, whereas Brazil yields a roughly 0.27 percent. The difference is not inconsequential because Brazil's percentage more than doubles Ecuador's. The mean of these percentages is 0.19. If this mean represents reality in some fashion and if South America has around 426 million people, the continent should have roughly 8.1 million autistic people.

The situation in Europe may be quantifiable. The organization Autism Europe estimates the incidence of ASD on the continent at roughly 1 percent. With a population of some 739 million people, Europe may have about 7.4 million autistic citizens.

Estimates in Asia cluster in East Asia, especially China, where perhaps 1 percent of the population has ASD. The incidence of ASD in South Korea, however, has been estimated at 2.6 percent. As in South America, these divergent numbers are difficult to reconcile. Complicating matters is the diversity of people and lands in Asia, which stretches from the Pacific Coast in the East to the eastern shores of the Mediterranean basin in the West. With these stipulations in mind, the mean of the percentages in China and South Korea is 1.8. If this mean and its extrapolation to all Asia are warranted, and Asia's population is roughly 4.5 billion, then it has some 810 million autistic citizens.

No less diverse than Asia, Africa poses perhaps the greatest challenges to the quantifier. The range of estimates in African countries is large. For example, estimates of the incidence of ASD in Nigeria, Tunisia and Egypt are 0.08 percent, 11.5 percent and 33.6 percent, respectively. Given such variations, an overall estimate is probably elusive so that the incidence of ASD in Africa cannot be guessed with any hope of precision. Further research is needed.

The case of Australia appears to be straightforward. In 2012 the Australian Bureau of Statistics estimated that some 115,400 Australians (0.5 percent) have ASD. The incidence of ASD in the rest of the world must rely on a World Health Organization estimate of 0.6 percent.

These numbers underscore the absence of global consensus about ASD's prevalence. The problem is unsurprising because scientists employ different research methodologies around the world. Moreover, ASD has not penetrated public consciousness to an equal degree everywhere, and not all nations fund robust research in ASD. It is also apparent that humans vary in a large number of ways. The reader cannot expect perfect unifor-mity to characterize a diverse species. Without uniformity, consensus is elusive.

ASD IN CHILDREN AND ADULTS

An ASD hallmark is early onset. Because the neurological underpin-nings of ASD tend to manifest themselves early in life, a diagnosis may confirm its presence in children by, and even before, age two. Early onset suggests that the biological factors governing the behaviors of an autistic child are in action almost from the beginning of life. Of course, it is diffi-cult to detect ASD before a child is old enough to display deficiencies in social interaction, but this factor does not mean that ASD is not present at the earliest stages in life, particularly if faulty genes cause ASD even if the environment mediates its severity.

A focus on children, however, risks obscuring the fact that not all cases of ASD receive prompt attention. Although the disorder is present very early, some people function well enough to evade detection until adult-hood. Hard data are elusive, but plenty of anecdotes, compiled by various organizations including National Public Radio, the psychiatry department at the University of North Carolina at Chapel Hill, and the Pennsylvania Bureau of Autism Services (PBAS), confirm that many autistic adults were undiagnosed during childhood and adolescence. Responding to a request from the PBAS in 2009, University of Pennsylvania associate professor of psychiatry and pediatrics David Mandell found that 14 of 141 patients at Norristown State Hospital (once known as the State Lunatic Hospital) in Norristown, Pennsylvania, likely had ASD but were undiagnosed or misdi-agnosed. The fact that ASD is incurable with current medical interven-tions proves that it must persist into adulthood. This persistence demands that autistic adults receive as much medical scrutiny as autistic children.

Persistence may manifest itself in several ways. For example, high func-tioning autistic adults may still have social deficits that impair their ability to function seamlessly at work and in social settings. Such adults may fit the legal criteria of disability even though they live independently and work.

Another classic ASD attribute is its prevalence among males. Research calculates that males are roughly five times more likely to be autistic than females. Attention has focused on the X chromosome, one of the sex chro-mosomes. It is thought that mutations (changes to the nucleotide bases that comprise genes and thus chromosomes) on the X chromosome cause or at least contribute to ASD. Males and females have different couplings of sex chromosomes. Human females have two X chromosomes whereas males have an X and Y chromosome. Because females have a pair of the

same sex chromosome (X), they must have a harmful mutation or mutations at the same place or places on both X chromosomes, an unlikely
event, for a girl or woman to be autistic. In males, however, the X chromosome attaches to the Y chromosome at only two places so that the genes on
the X chromosome may express themselves free from the influence of
almost all other genes, whereas in a woman, genes differently located on a
pair of X chromosomes do not function. In other words, a single harmful
mutation to a gene on an X chromosome may be expressed in males
whereas it would almost always be suppressed in females. Therefore, males
must more often be autistic than females. Incidentally this phenomenon is
not unique to ASD. The same rationale governs the fact that baldness is
more common in men than women.

CONCLUSION

Autism is best understood as a broad class of disorders (Autism Spectrum Disorder or ASD) that affects many areas of the body and that leads
to neurological, developmental, and behavioral deficits. ASD appears early
in life, even though some autistic people evade detection until adulthood.
It is much more common in males than females. Going beyond these
basics, the next chapter explores how our understanding of and attitudes
toward autism have evolved over time. In humans, the evolution of ideas,
attitudes, and other attributes is part of history.

2

The History of Autism Spectrum Disorder

The story of any significant movement or development is always large and complex. For this reason very few historical accounts can ever claim comprehensiveness. The same is true of any history of autism spectrum disorder (ASD). The history of ASD is largely an examination of ideas—scientific and medical concepts—and of the people who articulated and responded to them. This chapter cannot present every idea and person for fear that the story would never end. At best an examination of the most consequential ideas and people can be presented, thereby necessitating the omission of other important material. The list of readings at the end of this book augments the information here and in every other chapter.

THE EARLIEST HISTORY OF ASD

The attempt to understand a disease, malady, condition, affliction, ailment, or disorder by enumerating signs and symptoms, naming it, identifying and evaluating treatments, and performing kindred tasks has long been essential to medicine. ASD's story is no different. As discussed in chapter one, the word "autism" derives from an ancient Greek term, but it is important to remember that the Greeks never identified a disorder called autism or had any appreciation of a continuum of signs and symptoms essential to the modern understanding of ASD. Instead the history of ASD really begins in the twentieth century. An important part of this history dates to 1911, when Swiss psychiatrist Paul Eugen Bleuler coined the term "autism." In arriving at this term, he did not think that autism (or ASD, as it is classified today) was a unique disorder. That understanding would come later. Bleuler instead thought it part of a previously known mental disorder, schizophrenia. Bleuler concluded this because he thought that autism's signs and symptoms overlapped with those of schizophrenia. For example, schizophrenics may have social deficits, language impairment, and poor eye contact with others, which are signs and symptoms that usually appear in people with ASD.

Given such overlap, it is not surprising that Bleuler put ASD within the framework of schizophrenia. It is common for physicians, when they identify signs and symptoms, to search for an established disease or disorder for reference rather than invent a new category. This thinking, whose method is often summarized by the phrase "Ockham's razor," has roots in the philosophy of medieval Franciscan William of Ockham. Schizophrenia fit the bill because it was much on the mind of psychiatrists since German psychiatrist Emil Kraepelin had described its signs and symptoms in 1887. In fact Bleuler found it so interesting that he spent much of his career studying it and even coined the term "schizophrenia."

In this regard, note that both Kraepelin and Bleuler identified schizophrenia as a psychosis. Here the distinction between neurosis and psychosis is relevant. A neurosis is a type of abnormal coping mechanism. Anxiety, for example, may help a person cope with uncomfortable or unpleasant circumstances. There is probably no one alive today who has not felt anxious at one time or another. But when anxiety becomes so great or so pervasive that it impairs quality of life, it becomes a neurosis. Keep in mind that someone can be abnormally anxious or be otherwise neurotic without losing the ability to perceive reality more or less as most others do.

The matter is different with a psychosis, which distorts a person to the point of having an experience that differs greatly from the way most others perceive reality. Schizophrenia displays just such a distortion. A schizophrenic person, for example, might experience a hallucination. A man who sees his dead mother as though she were alive is experiencing just such a hallucination because his perception of his mother is untrue. He has broken from reality in a serious and alarming way, a theme Alfred Hitchcock explored in *Psycho*.

ASD EMERGES AS A UNIQUE DIAGNOSIS

ASD emerged as a unique diagnosis only when medical practitioners began to decide what it was not. ASD began to differentiate from related conditions in the late 1930s, when several researchers focused on the signs and symptoms that Bleuler had identified in 1911. Two conclusions deserve particular attention. First, scientists and medical practitioners distinguished ASD (which was then labeled simply autism) from what was then called mental retardation, but which might be thought a type of intellectual disability. The initial confusion between ASD and retardation stemmed from the fact that some people with ASD displayed cognitive deficits, which made easy their categorization as retarded. But ASD and retardation are not identical. The attempt to quantify intelligence, known as the intelligence quotient (IQ), highlighted the differences between ASD and retardation because scientists defined retardation as an IQ score no higher than 70 whereas those with ASD could display an IQ well above this number. It became clear therefore that people with ASD were not necessarily bound to the cognitive limitations that beset retardation.

The second conclusion weakened the judgment that ASD was a type of schizophrenia. The relationship between ASD and schizophrenia has always been difficult to pinpoint, and this chapter emphasizes that researchers have occasionally reasserted the connection between ASD and schizophrenia. But in the late 1930s a few scientists and physicians began to differentiate the two. The crucial factor was the realization that ASD and schizophrenia differed in timing. ASD researchers began to emphasize early childhood onset, whereas it was well known that schizophrenia tended to afflict people not in childhood but in early adulthood.

Concentration on ASD's early onset owes much to Austrian American physician Leo Kanner and Austrian pediatrician Johann "Hans" Asperger. Both focused their research on children and thus articulated and strengthened the conviction that ASD afflicts people early in life. Both had begun their research into what is now known as ASD in the 1930s. Asperger (1944) may have been the path breaker, but because Kanner published his seminal paper one year earlier (Kanner 1943) he usually receives priority. (Note the importance of priority to the sciences and medicine. For example, biologists and historians of science usually credit Charles Darwin with articulating the theory of evolution by natural selection because he was the first to publish even though his compatriot Alfred Russel Wallace had formulated the idea in the 1830s. True, Darwin had come to the same conclusions that decade, but only his publication in 1859 of *On the Origin of Species* thrust natural selection into the spotlight and ensured him priority. This reality is evident today in the fact that creationists never lash out at Wallace because Darwin is the target.)

Born in Austria, Leo Kanner, like many immigrants, made his mark in the United States, where he taught and conducted research at Johns Hopkins University in Baltimore, Maryland. Displaying literary gifts, Kanner initially wanted to be a writer, but his proficiency in the sciences and mathematics together with the realization that writing would not provide adequate income steered him toward medicine. Specializing in the diseases and disorders of children, Kanner came to understand autism in terms of social deficiencies. That is, he shifted the focus on ASD from cognition to socialization. In this way, Kanner broke from the preoccupation with IQ; this approach deemphasized the link between ASD and retardation even though this reframing of issues appears not to have been his intention. This step, to the extent that he was conscious of it, must have taken courage because the attempt to measure cognition was then very popular among social scientists. In his work, Kanner defined ASD primarily as an impediment to someone's ability to bond with others. Kanner emphasized that this hindrance surfaced very early in life, a perspective that lent itself to the inference that a person had ASD from birth to death.

Hans Asperger echoed many of these ideas, though it would be wrong to assume that he copied Kanner. Asperger conducted his own research and drew his own conclusions apart from Kanner even though it cannot be denied that he referenced and admired Kanner's work. Although Asperger noted many of the signs and symptoms that Kanner had articulated, he went beyond Kanner to emphasize that the children he studied often displayed marked intelligence. Calling these children "little professors," Asperger enthused about their ability to describe their interests in great detail. These children did not display cognitive impairment. Because he emphasized ASD's positive characteristics, Asperger was more optimistic about the condition than was Kanner. This optimism may have stemmed partly from political conditions. Asperger thought, lectured, and wrote when Nazism, nationalism, and authoritarianism in general, were ascendant in Europe. Because the Nazis brutalized the disabled, Asperger may have wanted to deemphasize aspects of disability in people with ASD to protect them from prejudice and loathing. In this context, Asperger was sympathetic to disabled people at a time when Germany and the United States felt such revulsion to them that these nations legalized the compulsory sterilization of such people in the belief that the disabled should not be permitted to pass their infirmity to offspring. U.S. Supreme Court justice Oliver Wendell Holmes Jr. encapsulated this view in his opinion in *Buck v. Bell* (1927).

Asperger was not vain and never attempted to attach his name to his life's work. That task fell to later generations of scientists and medical practitioners, who elevated him by naming Asperger's syndrome (sometimes referenced as Asperger syndrome) to honor his lifetime of achievements in child psychiatry. These scientists and medical practitioners assumed that Asperger's syndrome was not quite the same condition as autism, but current thinking, as discussed later in this chapters, has subsumed Asperger's syndrome into the larger classification of ASD.

DOUBTS EMERGE ABOUT THE UNIQUENESS OF ASD

In the 1940s, ASD took its first steps away from schizophrenia, but it did not venture far enough to gain autonomy. During the next decade, American neuropsychiatrist Lauretta Bender reconnected ASD and schizophrenia. Any account of a complex person will not do him or her justice, a truism that applies to Bender. She was not always popular. Critics thought her inflexible and imperious, as someone unwilling or unable to change her views even in the face of contrary evidence. Her friends found Bender far more accessible and willing to listen to diverse opinions. Sometimes even her avowed enemies softened their opinions after lengthy conversations with her. In any case, it seems clear that Bender did not reject others' ideas without a fair hearing. She was an avid reader of Kanner's work, though in crucial respects she disavowed his ideas.

Like Kanner and Asperger, Bender focused on children, though the similarities end here. Recall, in particular, Asperger's sympathy for autistic children. This generosity seems negligible in Bender, or at least less apparent than in Asperger. She understood the stark social and economic chasm that separated her from Kanner and Asperger. Kanner and Asperger had earned prestige and worked at elite institutions. Whether they intended it or not, they worked in a privileged setting and could confine their work only to patients whose parents could afford their treatment. Note, however, that neither abandoned the poor. Both were willing to accommodate desperate cases according to their own discretion. Bender had no such luxury because she worked at a state hospital that served as a place of last resort. Those who could not afford treatment anywhere else turned to Bender and her hospital.

Probably for this reason, Bender seems to have formed a sometimes unkind opinion of people. To her, ASD was no condition that could be tamed by tweaking a medicine or two, but was rather a full fledged psychosis that required aggressive treatment. As a psychosis, ASD must be, she thought, a form of schizophrenia. The problem, of course, was that schizophrenia was not thought to be a childhood malady. Bender responded that the type of schizophrenia (really ASD) that afflicted children differed from other forms of schizophrenia in its early onset. If schizophrenia really could afflict children, then Bender must have been right to reconnect ASD and schizophrenia, an idea that was discredited a decade earlier.

Dealing with psychosis, Bender could not be tepid. Her treatments, if bold, nevertheless flew in the face of conventional wisdom. Consensus held that electroshock therapy was too intensive to administer to children, and in the 1950s it was dangerous enough to traumatize adults. But Bender did not let these problems stop her, even though results were dismal. The children who received these treatments worsened. They often had to be institutionalized to the grief of parents. A sad episode involved Guy, the son of Jacqueline Susann, acclaimed author of the novel *Valley of the Dolls*. As usual Bender prescribed electroshock therapy for him even though he was just three years old. Afterwards Susann scarcely recognized her son, so listless was he. She had little choice but to institutionalize him, a decision that haunted her until death. Electroshock therapy was bad enough, but Bender compounded the problem by giving autistic children lysergic acid diethylamide (LSD), a drug that was controversial even in the 1950s. It often heightens anxiety, paranoia, and delusions. These effects are unsurprising because LSD derives from ergot, a fungus that may cause hallucinations when it infests foods. The medical literature decried this approach, but again Bender seems to have stiffened in the face of contrary winds. Perhaps more than anyone else in the 1950s, Bender caused thoughtful people to question the efficacy and safety of psychiatric treatments. The stigma against psychiatry appears to have lingered into the present.

THE EMERGENCE OF RIVAL PERSPECTIVES ABOUT ASD

Every facet of every person has its origin in biology, the environment, or a combination of the two. The emphasis on ASD's early onset in the work of Kanner, Asperger and Bender strongly suggests that biology must play some role in the malady's inception and severity. To be fair, Kanner was willing to consider environmental influences but he never gave them more than scant attention. Moreover, the fact that Kanner and Asperger had treated the children of affluent parents and Bender dealt with less affluent patients suggests that social and economic factors, both environmental, could not be strong in ASD because they varied so widely. Taken together, these components suggest that biology must play a crucial role in ASD. None of this evidence eliminates environmental factors, though the medical practitioner might infer that such factors are unimportance.

Given this context, it may seem surprising that Austrian psychoanalyst Bruno Bettelheim expended so much energy redefining ASD in environmental terms. He took pains to single out parents, especially mothers, as the culprits of ASD in their children. Bettelheim believed that cold, distant parents, especially mothers, failed to bond with their children, thus causing ASD in them. In his view, the absence of nurturing was the villain in ASD. Here was the foundation for the term "refrigerator mom." Bettelheim faced opposition. Critics held that he was an imposter who tried to pass off others' ideas as his own. The charge of plagiarism, if true, can cost a physician his or her medical license. Bettelheim's reputation did not survive, and if Bender's behavior soured people's views of psychiatry, Bettelheim's apparent unscrupulousness only heightened the perception that psychiatry was not an honorable profession.

Parallel to these developments was the work of British psychiatrist Eleanor Mildred Creak. A confidant of Bender, Creak reinforced the perception that ASD was a psychosis. In many other ways, however, she departed from Bender's views. In making her case, Creak opposed Bettelheim's focus on the environment in the form of parenting. Refrigerator moms did not cause ASD. The problem was primarily and perhaps wholly genetic. Here was a robust statement that biology plays not merely the leading role in ASD but possibly the only role. Departing from the sentiment that autistic children required institutionalization, Creak stressed that outpatient care could be effective and that institutionalization should be the last resort. A convert to the Society of Friends (Quakers), Creak established a reputation for compassionate care. Her attempt to humanize the treatment of children with ASD came at a crucial moment when many thoughtful people, put off by the work of Bender and Bettelheim, distrusted psychiatry.

REVIVAL OF ASD AS A UNIQUE DIAGNOSIS

Amid this bustle, Kanner continued to influence ASD's study. In the 1960s he was central to a campaign to reestablish ASD's uniqueness. This position stemmed from Kanner's conviction that ASD was primarily a neurological condition, one unique from other such disturbances. Yet he was no biological determinist, focusing throughout his career on the role of parenting. Earlier was noted the tendency to blame parents for ASD in their children because of their failure to nurture. Kanner had also articulated this premise in his 1943 article. In the aftermath of this criticism, parents around the world organized against the implication that they caused ASD in their offspring. These groups emphasized parental affection in insisting that the refrigerator mom thesis was a grotesque caricature.

The idea that ASD was a unique disorder gained strength from the work of German psychologist Beate Hermelin and her colleague, British psychologist Neil O'Connor. In 1970, the two published the first in a series of papers on the abilities of children with ASD known as savants. The term "savant" derives from the Latin *sapere*, meaning "to be wise." In the strictest sense, a savant is a learned scholar. In popular culture, the term "savant" has come to mean anyone with an astonishing mental talent. In this context, a savant might be a person capable of completing a three hour mathematics test in twenty minutes, or a person with an exceptionally retentive memory. In such circumstances it is difficult to conclude that such a person is necessarily brilliant. For example, a savant might memorize pi (roughly 3.14) to an astounding number of decimal places while at the same time being unable to read a train schedule. Hermelin and O'Connor used the term "savant" to denote children with such abilities, even when such children displayed cognitive deficits. The fact that these savants were remarkable in striking ways strengthened the thought that ASD must be unique, at least in this capacity.

The case for uniqueness gained further traction from the work of British child psychiatrist Michael Rutter, a man who has shaped ASD research to a degree that invites comparison with Kanner and Asperger. Mindful of Kanner's work, Rutter strengthened the sentiment that ASD was a neurological condition. He based this conclusion on his work to document the connection between ASD and epilepsy, noting that some epileptics are autistic. Because epilepsy is a neurological condition, ASD must also be one. A focus on neurology suggests that ASD originates in biology, namely in the genes. In this context, researchers must enlarge their knowledge of genetics.

RELATIONSHIP BETWEEN GENETICS AND ASD

The science of genetics, originating in the work of nineteenth-century Austrian monk and naturalist Gregor Mendel, has influenced medicine and all the sciences in profound ways. ASD's study benefits from this focus, though not all medical practitioners agree on the role of genes in ASD.

A basic insight governs the application of genetics to a variety of phenomena: the more genes two organisms share the more traits they share, with the converse also being true. In ASD's context, genetic studies have centered on people who share large numbers of genes, namely close biological relations. The study of siblings has been central to this approach. In studying siblings, researchers have assumed that a person with ASD is more likely to have a sibling with ASD than is a non-ASD person to have sibling with ASD. The attempt to quantify an event's likelihood lies in the domain of probability. In the contexts of ASD and probability, quantification is not easy because a researcher cannot guess how prevalent ASD should be among siblings. Moreover, the number of genes that two siblings share cannot be known precisely, though the mean of all possibilities should be fifty, the odds of turning up heads in a coin toss. Only the application of statistical tests can determine whether a particular incidence of ASD among siblings is significant. The meaning of the word "significant" is itself a statistical construct.

The use of statistics is thus crucial to ASD's study. British psychiatrist Michael Rutter has long advocated the importance of statistical tests. A proponent of biology as a large factor in the incidence and severity of ASD, Rutter might have been expected to favor a genetic cause of ASD. At first, however, Rutter had doubts because only about two percent of people with ASD had a sibling with ASD, a rate that he judged too low to be significant. Yet by 1968 Rutter had changed course upon realizing that even a two percent linkage was much higher than in the general population. That is, people with ASD have, according to statistical tests, significantly more siblings with ASD than do people without ASD.

Behavioral geneticists were also doubters initially, but their position was tenuous given the difficulty in establishing the genetic causes of behavior. The focus on behavior complicated rather than clarified the relationship between genetics and ASD, leading other researchers to avoid behavioral studies. Note that genetics may be divided into hard (physical) and soft (behavioral) components. Whether a cyclist has a long or short nose (a physical trait) does not deter him from accosting anyone who endangers him on the road (a behavior). Should the cyclist get close enough he will fight the reckless driver (an extension of the original behavior), during which a punch to the face may break his nose (a modification of the physical trait). Therefore the division into hard and soft components is more instructive than real.

The role of genetics in ASD gained traction as researchers articulated the idea that many genes must be responsible for its severity. This approach was novel in a way because Mendel had focused only on the action of single genes or at most a pair of genes. Yet the idea that multiple genes control a trait was gaining adherents in a variety of fields, and it seemed natural to invoke this mechanism to explain ASD's severity. Briefly, if someone has only a small number of genes that govern the onset and severity of ASD, his or her condition should be mild. If, however, an individual has a large number of such harmful genes, his or her condition should be severe. The notion that multiple genes govern ASD thus explains the phenomenon of a spectrum, meaning that severity of symptoms varies over a broad continuum because the number of harmful genes a person might inherit varies widely.

MOVEMENT TOWARD RECOGNITION THAT ASD IS A SPECTRUM OF DISORDERS

Such thinking has underpinned the modern understanding of ASD that has emerged from a variety of scientific and medical studies. As early as 1968, Canadian psychologist Victor Lotter emphasized that people with ASD do not necessarily manifest all ASD's signs and symptoms. Such thinking was another way of expressing the notion that ASD varied in severity from person to person and so was consistent with a multi-genetic interpretation of ASD.

The emphasis on variations in ASD's severity found favor in other quarters. Even researchers who envisioned ASD as a psychosis, and who were thus inclined to focus on its excesses, conceded that not all cases of ASD were severe. The existence of mild cases confirmed that ASD must vary in severity. At the same time, British psychiatrist Lorna Wing, writing in the 1980s, began to seek unity by emphasizing commonalities between autism and Asperger's syndrome. If these seemingly separate conditions were related, then ASD must include a broad range of signs, symptoms, prognoses, treatments, and outcomes.

Aware of these factors, the 2013 edition of the *Diagnostic Statistical Manual of Mental Disorders* reorganized the medical understanding of ASD in important ways. Perhaps the most significant change was abandonment of the term "autism" in favor of autism spectrum disorder (ASD). If ASD were a continuum, then perpetuation of Asperger's syndrome as a separate condition was no longer justified. What had been designated Asperger's syndrome was really a set of comparatively mild signs and symptoms on the ASD continuum. This logic applied to other conditions. Pervasive developmental disorder not otherwise specified, a condition that had been thought to be related to but distinct from classical autism and Asperger's syndrome, was likewise subsumed into the larger framework of ASD. Similar conditions, notably childhood disintegrative disorder and Rett syndrome, also disappeared as separate diagnoses in favor of incorporation into ASD. ASD emerged as an umbrella under which are grouped several conditions once considered separate. In sum, the current emphasis is on unification rather than fragmentation.

MOVEMENT TOWARD RECOGNITION THAT ASD IS A DISABILITY

Disability is a sensitive issue because stigma sometimes mars it, impeding disabled people from asserting their rights by seeking legal protection of their status. The reality of ASD reinforces this truth because a person with ASD may not appear to be disabled in an obvious way. For example, a person confined to a wheelchair because of paralyzed legs is obviously disabled, but the able-bodied person with ASD displays no such evident infirmity. Society's expectation is that any able-bodied person, with ASD or not, should work rather than claim a disability.

Given these circumstances, ASD has not always been classified a disability. Even today a person is not disabled by virtue of having ASD. In 2017 the U.S. Social Security Administration clarified its rules governing ASD. For a person with ASD to qualify for disability payments, his or her medical records must meet three criteria. First, a medical practitioner must document the person's social deficits. Second, the medical records must document the person's deficits in communication, both verbal and nonverbal. Third, a medical practitioner must document that the person displays repetitive behaviors, interests, or activities.

In this context, note that a person with ASD may qualify for disability benefits at any stage in life. True, most diagnoses are made in childhood, but someone who has avoided detection until adulthood and who meets the three criteria is not barred from benefits just because he or she did not have them as a child. These comments aside, the circumstances for receipt of disability benefits differ for children and adults. By virtue of their status, children receive benefits in the form of Supplemental Security Income (SSI). SSI, however, is available only to families with limited income and assets. That is, the program is means tested. An adult, on the other hand, may qualify for Social Security Disability Insurance (SSDI), but these benefits are available only to someone who has amassed a sufficiently long work history. An adult with ASD who has not worked cannot qualify for SSDI. In this case SSI is the lone possibility.

As a disabled person, someone with ASD is protected by Americans with Disabilities Act (ADA). In 1990, Congress enacted this law to extend the protections of civil rights legislation to disabled people. Explicit in the law is the prohibition against discrimination in all areas of the economy and civil society. Any venue open to the public must extend these protections to all disabled people. An important ADA provision requires employers and businesses to make reasonable accommodations for disabled people so that they experience no discrimination. The U.S. Equal Employment Opportunity Commission mandates that all employers with at least fifteen workers obey the ADA. The Federal Communications Commission enforces the compliance of telecommunications firms, including any business that operates online. Other government agencies enforce other aspects of the ADA. In 2008 Congress amended the ADA to clarify the definition of disability, an action that has not weakened any ADA protection for people with ASD and other disabilities.

MOVEMENT TOWARD PUBLIC AWARENESS OF ASD

Since the 1980s, public awareness of ASD has increased as activists and people with ASD have raised its profile. No study can name all participants in this movement, but luminaries in Hollywood, literature, and the media have played a significant role in heightening awareness. Several movies have examined ASD, perhaps none more movingly than *Rain Man*. In 1988 acclaimed director Barry Levinson produced the movie, though its motive force was celebrated actor Dustin Hoffman, who had nurtured the concept years before Levinson entered the project. In the movie, Hoffman played Raymond Babbitt, a man with ASD who had considerable social deficits but a remarkable memory. Here was the type of savant that medical practitioners had studied. Critics praised the film, which won numerous awards including the Academy Awards for best picture, best actor, best original screenplay, and best director. *Rain Man* triumphed at least partly because it allowed audiences to sympathize with the deficits and abilities of man with ASD.

In literature, nonfiction is an important vehicle for advancing public awareness about ASD. Particularly important have been contributions from authors with ASD. Foremost among them is Temple Grandin, an American livestock scientist. In her books, articles, and essays, Grandin has described the difficulties that led medical practitioners to doubt her ability ever to function in society. Despite these opinions, Grandin's mother never wavered in her devotion. This support helped Grandin transcend her situation. She earned a PhD in animal science from the University of Illinois, a respected land grant university, in Champaign-Urbana. An authority on the design and operation of livestock buildings, Grandin has emerged as a notable author and lecturer. Her numerous honors include induction into the prestigious American Academy of Arts and Sciences in Cambridge, Massachusetts. Her successes demonstrate that people with ASD can achieve prominence.

More generally, the media have heightened public awareness about ASD. Over the years, radio, television, and print and online journalism have profiled people with ASD, telling their stories in compelling ways. The effect has been to humanize those with ASD and to create empathy for them. True, some stories seek sensationalism, but reputable journalists have featured people with ASD in realistic and sympathetic terms. These efforts are so numerous that a September 2017 Google search with the phrase "stories about autism" yielded more than 23 million results.

Yet media attention has not always been beneficial. For example, chapter 9 examines the claims of a cadre of physicians and scientists and a handful of celebrities that some vaccines cause ASD. These beliefs emerged from faulty and biased research that purported to link vaccination to a supposedly new type of ASD. In its reporting, most of the media acted too rashly to be objective, knocking over the dominoes that led to uncritical coverage of this research and to the conclusion that celebrities' opinions were newsworthy in this instance. The celebrities had no medical training and could not evaluate research that claimed to link vaccinations and ASD. Consequently these stories were more sensationalism than journalism.

CONCLUSION

ASD's history emphasizes the initial tendency to group its signs and symptoms within the older framework of schizophrenia. Separation was not easy to achieve, and as late as the 1950s some researchers maintained that what is now called ASD was really part of schizophrenia. Another complicating factor has been the nature versus nurture debate, scrutinized in the next chapter. In particular, the claim that refrigerator moms cause ASD in their children put parents on the defensive and created a backlash. Meanwhile other researchers focused on the role of biology, particularly genetics, in determining ASD's onset and severity. An important trend has been the growing awareness that ASD is not a monolith but instead a broad continuum of signs and symptoms that reflect the multiplicity of disorders under one umbrella. These developments have not occurred in a vacuum. As all facets of society have become more aware of ASD, people with ASD have been able to seek protection from various government agencies and laws, including the U.S. Social Security Administration and the ADA. The focus on faulty genes as determiners of ASD expands in chapter 3, which examines causes and risk factors.

REFERENCES

Asperger, Hans. Trans. 1944; trans. 1991. "'Autistic Psychopathy' in Childhood." In *Autism and Asperger Syndrome*. Edited and translated by Uta Frith, 37–92. Cambridge, UK: Cambridge University Press.

Buck v. Bell, 274 U.S. 200 (1927).

Kanner, Leo. 1943. "Autistic Disturbances of Affective Contact." *The Nervous Child* 2:217–250.

3

Causes and Risk Factors

Central to the practice of medicine is the attempt to identify the causes and risk factors of a disease, condition, malady, affliction, ailment, or disorder. Sometimes a cause or risk factor can be known with such precision that doubt is impossible. For example, no responsible physician would deny that yellow fever virus causes the tropical disease yellow fever or that obesity is a risk factor for some cancers, diabetes, and heart disease. Although autism spectrum disorder (ASD) is a complex disorder and although debate continues about its causes and risk factors, evidence is growing that these causes and factors have their origin in biology, namely in the genes. Chapter 2 emphasized that debate and varying perspectives are integral to ASD's history. Even if its causes and risk factors remain open to discussion, they must have roots in biology, the environment, or a combination of the two, as discussed in chapter 2. Here the connections between these categories are explored. The treatment of biological and environmental factors may be easiest to grasp if each is considered in turn, in a nature versus nurture format. Separate treatment of these issues in this chapter does not mean that they work separately in anyone. Biology and the environment go hand in hand in defining every human being.

NATURE VERSUS NURTURE

The study of ASD's causes and risk factors is part of a broad debate over the roles of nature and nurture. Nature refers to biological forces, whereas nurture encompasses environmental factors. In this book the term "biology" refers to purely physical and chemical properties; "environment" refers to the interaction of an organism, a person in this case, with the world that exists outside it. For example, while biology has given the human brain sufficient complexity to understand abstract concepts, such understanding seems to occur only as the result of people's interaction with specific elements of the environment. For convenience such interactions will be labeled as learning.

Desire for the clearest definitions of biology and the environment should not obscure the fact that both interact. For example, a Caucasian person who lives in the temperate zone may have pale skin in winter. This baseline condition is under biological (genetic) control. In the summer, however, exposure to intense sunlight may darken his or her skin, sometimes markedly. The interaction between sunlight and skin is an environmental process that modifies the baseline condition so that biology and the environment interact to produce the final skin color. This sequence characterizes all biology-environment outcomes.

Concern over biological and environmental factors has shaped the understanding of ASD. Chapter 2 stated that ASD's biological causes and risk factors originate in the genes. On the other hand, the refrigerator mom thesis seeks a completely environmental understanding of ASD by supposing that parents, especially mothers, cause ASD in their child or children by failing to nurture them. According to this thinking, failure to nurture and to bond with children causes their marked social deficits, as is evident in numerous people with ASD. Note that this reasoning requires that interactions between parents and children be entirely a social exercise lacking any biological considerations. For convenience and to begin sorting out gene-environment factors, the next section focuses on genetics.

GENETICS

Chapter 3 discussed the origins of genetics in nineteenth-century Austrian monk and naturalist Gregor Mendel's life and work. Mendel never used the term "gene" but instead thought in terms of particles that parents passed to their offspring. This insight remains valid today, though scientists now conceptualize these particles as large molecules. Although overlooked during his lifetime, possibly because he published so little, Mendel made a fundamental contribution to knowledge because the study of genes is central to any understanding of life. This is so because genes direct the synthesis of chemicals known as proteins, which may be assembled into any and every structure in the body. That is, genes contain the instructions or blueprint that builds the physical details of every organism, including a person.

These genes must be copied whenever a cell divides. Because cells die, continuous reiteration of the genes is essential to all life, which would perish unless it retained the genes (in the form of copies) inherited at conception. But this copying is not always perfect. Imperfections in copying are known as mutations. A mutation is a chemical change to a nucleotide base, a large molecule that may be envisioned as a building block of a gene. A single nucleotide base is part of a larger molecule known as deoxyribose nucleic acid (DNA) or of its companion molecule known as ribose nucleic acid (RNA). Each human cell contains all the nucleotide bases (all the DNA) necessary to direct its activity. (By contrast a virus may be made up of either DNA or RNA, so that generalities do not apply to all life.) For convenience, scientists have labeled the nucleotide bases. In DNA they are adenine, guanine, cytosine, and thymine. These bases are the same in RNA except that uracil replaces thymine. These bases align in a definite order to form genes, meaning that the order determines the identity and function of that gene. One nucleotide base never suffices to build a gene. Although the number of nucleotide bases in any one gene is unique, the total number when all are summed is enormous. In a single human cell that number is roughly 3 billion.

A mutation may be small, as in the deletion or addition of a single carbon atom to a nucleotide base, granting the reality that no carbon atom is unbonded in any plant or animal cell. Alternatively, a mutation may be large, as in the deletion or addition of an entire nucleotide base to a gene. Most mutations are harmful because seldom is a chemical change just the right type to benefit an organism. Beneficial mutations do occur but are extremely rare.

The centrality of genes to every biological process has led many scientists and medical practitioners to seek ASD's causes and risk factors in a person's genes. This line of thought bears fruit in the cases of fragile X syndrome, Rett syndrome, and tuberous sclerosis complex, all now recognized as being on the autism spectrum. Not every instance of fragile X syndrome, Rett syndrome, or tuberous sclerosis complex represents a case of ASD. Likewise, not every person with ASD has one of these conditions. In other words, these conditions and ASD sometimes overlap such that some instances of the three are manifestations of ASD and some cases of ASD are the three genetic conditions.

Fragile X syndrome afflicts the X chromosome. The X chromosome is a sex chromosome of which both human males and human females have at least one, and it (like all chromosomes) is comprised of genes. That is, a focus on the X chromosome, or any chromosome for that matter, leads researchers to concentrate on genes.

The culprit in fragile X syndrome is a single gene with too many nucleotide bases, doubtless the result of one or more mutations. Regarding this syndrome, the faulty gene has three extra nucleotide bases, namely cytosine, guanine, and guanine in that order. These extra nucleotide bases impair the gene's functions, analogous to the reality that extra air in a tire distorts it so that blowouts are more probable. The gene's impairments cause cognitive deficits, a condition that was formerly known as mental retardation. Remember that ASD can also reduce cognition. Researchers have demonstrated that about 15 to 30 percent of people with ASD have this faulty gene, though only about 1 to 3 percent of girls and women have it, linking the gene to the X chromosome. This outcome is inevitable because the disorder under consideration is fragile X syndrome; boys and men should display it more often than girls and women because males have X and Y sex chromosomes. These chromosomes, being different, do not pair except at the two points where they connect. Genes on the X chromosome (and the Y for that matter)—helpful or harmful—express themselves, provided they are active, without influence from another gene because they are unpaired. In fact, researchers have uncovered the expected results, estimating that roughly 1 in 3,600 males and 1 in 8,000 females have the faulty gene. These numbers may seem tiny, but keep in mind that fragile X syndrome is the most common form of inherited mental deficiency. On top of mental impairment, fragile X syndrome leads many sufferers to display the social deficits that have long been a hallmark of ASD. What is clear to medical researchers is that fragile X syndrome and ASD are linked.

Rett syndrome likewise afflicts a gene on the X chromosome and so, like fragile X syndrome, affects more females than males. Affecting just 1 in 10,000 to 15,000 females, Rett syndrome is less common than fragile X syndrome but is no less consequential. The affliction may deform the head, stop the brain from reaching normal size (microcephaly), cause seizures, sleep apnea, and hyperventilation, and impair development of fine motor skills. (Microcephaly always impairs cognition in humans; this book entertains no hypotheses about cognition in *Homo floresiensis* [Flores Man], who once inhabited the Indonesian island of Flores.) Medical researchers once estimated that as many as two-fifths of girls with Rett syndrome have ASD. Today, however, the inclusion of Rett syndrome on the autism spectrum means that every case of it is also an instance of ASD so that ASD completely subsumes it. But keep in mind that not every case, indeed not most cases, of ASD is an instance of Rett syndrome.

The third condition, tuberous sclerosis complex, is an autosomal dominant disorder. Unlike fragile X syndrome and Rett syndrome, tuberous sclerosis complex does not affect a sex chromosome but rather a nonsex chromosome, known as an autosome. All humans have 23 pairs (or 46) chromosomes. Only a single pair are sex chromosomes whereas all the rest are autosomes. Tuberous sclerosis complex results from a mutation to two autosomal genes, meaning that it can harm any of the remaining 22 pairs of chromosomes. Because tuberous sclerosis complex is a dominant disorder, it necessarily damages a dominant gene.

In his pioneering work, Mendel introduced the concepts of dominance and recessiveness. He noted after several years of experiments with the garden pea that genes must align in pairs and that a gene must have different versions in the way that toothbrushes come in different versions or kinds. Taking this analogy a stride forward, different versions of a gene have different arrangements of the same nucleotide bases just as the bristles in a toothbrush may be removed, shuffled randomly, and reinserted in the original holes.

The order of nucleotide bases is not the lone variable to consider because at the macrolevel, some versions of a gene may be dominant whereas another version may be recessive. If a version is dominant, it will always be expressed even when only one gene in a pair is of this type. In contrast a recessive version of a gene will never express itself unless both genes in a pair are of this type. It might help to think of the relationship between a dominant version of a gene and a recessive version as a type of power exchange in which the dominant version, when it is present in a pair, will always mask or overpower the recessive version. Because a dominant version of a gene is always expressed when paired with a recessive version, a harmful mutation on a dominant gene will always injure an organism. For this reason, by any medical accounting tuberous sclerosis complex is comparatively widespread, afflicting about 1 in 6,000 people.

With this as background, it is obvious that tuberous sclerosis complex must impair the body in several ways, one being diminution of its cells' ability to synthesize proteins. Recall that protein synthesis is under genetic control and that the two autosomal mutations no longer are efficient so that they ineptly direct processes like protein synthesis and assemblage into the body's structures. The situation is akin to a blueprint with numerous errors that impede a building's construction.

Results can be dire because tuberous sclerosis complex causes physical problems like skin lesions and seizures, as well as mental deficiencies. Social impairments are also marked and align with the classic deficits seen in people with ASD. The overlap between tuberous sclerosis and ASD is large, with perhaps one quarter of all children who have tuberous sclerosis complex exhibiting signs and symptoms of ASD; but only about 4 percent of all children with ASD have tuberous sclerosis complex, reinforcing the fact that not every case of ASD is an instance of tuberous sclerosis complex.

THE ENVIRONMENT

With the preceding information in mind, it is unsurprising that several medical researchers favor a genetic cause of ASD. Even if this approach is correct, it does not mean that environmental factors must be inconsequential. The environment also appears to contribute to ASD's severity if not to its onset. Our task here is to pinpoint the most important environmental factors. This book acknowledges the probability that ASD is under genetic control. In grappling with the relationship between genetics and the environment, consider a military analogy whereby genes provide the ammunition for a gun and the environment contributes to the gun's rate and range of firing.

Another way to conceive both the differences between biology and the environment and their interactions is through the terms "genotype" and "phenotype." Your genotype is the totality of all the genes you inherited from your parents. You have many genes even though only a small number are active. That means only a small number are expressed, or "turned on." These genes determine your physical attributes, known as your phenotype. Moving beyond the phenotype, the sum of all genes in a person is his or her genotype, though the word "genotype" may be defined in terms of the species in addition to the individual. Here again, isolation of genotype from phenotype is impossible because the environment influences the expression of genes. To reiterate, the environment shapes the physical traits that define the phenotype. Because ASD is part of the phenotype (in addition to being an outcome of the genotype), the environment must help trigger genes to establish ASD's severity, even though its onset appears to be purely a genetic phenomenon.

In terms of the environment, the refrigerator mom thesis needs no additional commentary and no longer has credibility among medical professionals. Nonetheless some parental factors must shape ASD's severity if not its onset. These factors diverge from the refrigerator mom thesis by not blaming parental styles for ASD. Rather than a focus on warmth and nurturing, or their absence, current research emphasizes the role of aging and other biological aspects by noting, among other phenomena, that as both mother and father age, their chances of having a child with ASD increase. This information expresses ASD's environmental burdens in biological terms.

Taking the parents one at a time, eleven published studies between 2001 and 2009 examined the relationship between the mother's age and her likelihood of having a child with ASD. These studies yielded similar findings. Briefly, a pregnant woman is not at great risk of delivering a baby with ASD if she is age 35 and younger. Above this age, however, the odds turn against her so that she is roughly 50 percent more likely than a younger woman to have a baby with ASD. This risk seems to be constant above age

35, so that a 36-year-old woman and a woman who is ten years older are both at roughly the same risk of delivering a baby with ASD, even though neither is at significantly greater risk compared to a woman below age 35.

The problem with advanced longevity is that a woman's eggs age along with her. As these eggs age their quality deteriorates with the result that developmental deficits of various kinds may beset the baby, deficits that are not limited to ASD. Older women are also more likely to have a child with Down syndrome or certain other types of cognitive and lifespan impairments. The case of Down syndrome may be significant in this context because it arises from the child's inheritance of an extra autosome. That is, the problem is linked to a chromosome (in this case an autosome) just as fragile X syndrome, Rett syndrome, and tuberous sclerosis complex all involve chromosomal defects. Remember that a problem with a gene is at the same time a problem with a chromosome because genes make up chromosomes.

Advanced age may usher in additional problems for mothers, including a diminishing capacity to regulate the production of hormones necessary to ensure proper development of a fertilized egg. Recall that a hormone is a type of chemical messenger that signals a part of the body to synthesize or regulate the production of another chemical to hasten or delay some process. For example, a hormone directs the implantation of a fertilized egg in the uterus. Without such a chemical messenger a fertilized egg cannot implant to initiate the nine-month gestation necessary to transform it into a viable baby.

The problem of advanced age in fathers appears to result from a greater rate of mutations to genes in the sperm. Here the degree of risk is comparable, but not the same as, the risk to older women. Recall that women above age 35 have a greater risk of delivering a baby with ASD than do women under age 35. In men the threshold appears to be age 40, after which the likelihood of fathering a child with ASD increases by more than 50 percent. This risk is not constant as is the case with older women. As men age the risk of fathering an autistic child rises steeply so that a 50-year-old man bears more than twice the risk than does a man under age 40.

Keep in mind that aging occurs within the framework of environmental factors. That said, aging is a biological phenomenon that appears to be malleable in relation to some environmental factors. Recall that as a man ages the number of mutations to genes in the sperm increases. If this increase is solely the result of biology, then the environment is irrelevant. But researchers have established that environmental factors, like exposure to toxins, can increase the rate of mutations. It follows, therefore, that if mutations to the genes in the sperm can result from such factors, then the environment must play some role in ASD's onset and severity, even though not all environmental factors appear to influence onset.

Other risk factors go beyond parental age, centering on the timing of birth and the newborn's size and weight. Research demonstrates that babies born after a normal gestation of nine months are least likely to have ASD. But gestations shorter than nine months necessarily yield a preterm baby, often known as a premature baby. Prematurity is itself an ASD risk factor that coincides with two other factors: low birth weight and small-ness. These factors are related because a premature baby has not completed a full nine months of development necessary to grow sufficiently large and heavy. The greater the deviation from a normal gestation, the greater is the risk that the baby will have ASD.

Several factors linked to the mother's health affect gestation. Mothers whose health is not optimal are at risk of having a child with ASD. Common maternal problems that lead to prematurity, low birth weight, and smallness, and thus potentially to ASD include high blood pressure and diabetes. Research has documented, among other factors, the risk that cigarette smoking poses to mothers and their babies, including prematurity, low birth weight and small size, and ASD because of these factors.

Other environmental factors affect mother and developing child. For example, a woman who conceives a child within a year of having the previous baby increases the risk that this second child will have ASD. On the other hand, evidence suggests that women who take vitamin and mineral supplements during pregnancy may lower the risk of bearing a child with ASD, though this conclusion does not appear to support the consumption of massive amounts of vitamins and minerals, a practice known as mega dosing. Current research focuses on many nutrients, among them folic acid. This B vitamin appears to reduce the risk that a child will develop ASD when an expectant mother supplements her diet with it. Good sources of folic acid include spinach, citrus fruits, and beans. Expectant mothers—and everyone for that matter—should base their nutrition on advice from a physician or other medical expert.

Additional environmental factors linking mother and fetus include the finding that obesity may put a pregnant woman at risk for delivering a baby with ASD. Moreover, women who take certain antidepressants during the first trimester of pregnancy appear to be at risk of having a baby with ASD. Caution should be exercised whenever antidepressants may confer greater benefits than risks. In addition, pregnant women who control their fevers with aspirin or another fever reducers appear to be at less risk of having an baby with ASD than expectant mothers who do not take medicine to control their fevers. A baby born with ASD appears to develop less severe signs and symptoms when the mother breastfeeds him or her. Conversely, the sooner a child is weaned off breast milk the greater appears to be the risk of worsening his or her ASD.

Another possible environmental factor pivots upon the debate over mercury contaminated fish. It is well established that the metal mercury is toxic when humans consume it. It should follow that consumption of fish containing mercury is hazardous. In many respects this inference is sound, but it is not proven that consumption of such fish increases the risk that a pregnant woman will have a baby with ASD. Given these circumstances it is difficult to determine whether the benefits of eating fish outweigh concerns that mercury in fish might harm a developing fetus and thereby worsen conditions like ASD.

Beyond these considerations, the use of drugs, even prescribed ones, may be an important environmental factor. Part of pharmacology's history is the replacement of traditional home therapies with synthetic drugs, but these medicines can exacerbate problems or cause new ones. This situation applies to ASD, where a suite of medicines has increased its incidence. Notorious has been thalidomide, which physicians sometimes prescribed to expectant mothers in the 1950s and 1960s. It is now evident that the drug causes birth defects. Given in the first trimester of pregnancy, thalidomide sharply increases the risk that the baby will display ASD's signs and symptoms.

A second drug is misoprostol, given to treat stomach ulcers. Research in Brazil has demonstrated that expectant mothers who take the drug increase the danger that their baby will have ASD. In a similar category is valproic acid. Pregnant women who take it expose their unborn child to a range of birth defects. The earlier its use in pregnancy the greater is the risk that the baby will have ASD.

Another peril is the viral infection rubella. Symptoms may be mild, though pregnant women who catch the virus incur the risk of delivering a baby with ASD. This risk is highest when the expectant mother contracts the disease within eight weeks after conception, when she may still be unaware of her pregnancy and not seek medical treatment.

In another class of environmental dangers are certain insecticides. Since the 1940s the use of insecticides in various settings has generated controversy. These chemicals are toxins by design. Attention now focuses on organophosphates, a class of insecticides that replaced dichlorodiphenyltrichloroethane (DDT). Many scientists once thought organophosphates were safer than DDT when accidentally exposed to humans. However, this thought has proven incorrect as exposure to these insecticides can damage the central nervous system (CNS) and thereby cause attention deficits, hyperactivity, and ASD in children. The problem cannot here receive coverage beyond the statement that several scientific and agricultural developments make organophosphates particularly appealing to farmers. Given this reality, it seems reasonable to fear an increase in ASD diagnoses.

Other critics have focused on the administration of vaccines to children. Consult chapter 9 for the details of this controversy. Here it suffices to emphasize that faulty science and the opinions of uninformed celebrities caused widespread fears that vaccines might cause ASD in children. Fury surrounded an old version of a vaccine that conferred immunity against measles, mumps, and rubella (MMR). MMR vaccines have been and continue to be part of modern medicine. Responsible journalism and science have since proven these fears groundless, but for a time the public fretted over whether to vaccinate their children.

A complex case is oxytocin because it does not fit neatly into nature versus nurture calculations. On the nature side of the equation, the brain's hypothalamus produces oxytocin, whose effects can be striking because it seems to cement familial bonds. Moreover, its presence during orgasm may contribute to the post climax tenderness shared by a couple. Furthermore, the hypothalamus increases oxytocin levels late in pregnancy because it stimulates labor contractions. The chemical is also an environmental factor because a nurse or obstetrician/gynecologist may administer it to a woman to strengthen weak contractions. Yet such women are at risk of delivering a baby with ASD. In these instances, the baby may develop marked social deficits even when physical problems are absent. More research is necessary for medical practitioners to gain a fuller understanding of the relationship between oxytocin and ASD.

Another important environmental factor concerns oxygen's role in a fetus. All aerobic respiration, including that of humans, demands oxygen such that aerobic organisms cannot survive without it. The need for oxygen is lifelong and begins in the womb. Sufficient oxygen is necessary in every aspect of a fetus' development. The brain in particular needs an ample supply for normal development, without which the risk of developing ASD increases.

These factors affect a fetus. After birth, fewer environmental factors appear to be relevant. Nonetheless some aspects of the environment may steer a child toward ASD as late as age two. The most significant factors appear to be interaction with other children and outdoor activity. Children who seldom communicate with their peers or play outdoors appear to be at risk of ASD. Such a child must already have ASD, which limited communication and outdoor activities worsen.

In recounting her life, Temple Grandin, the American livestock expert mentioned in chapter 2, cites other environmental factors in her childhood, the most consequential being her mother's expectation that Grandin excel and her rejection of the doctors' pessimism. Grandin believes that these actions and beliefs, both environmental, minimized her ASD.

GENETIC AND ENVIRONMENTAL FACTORS

The interplay between biology and the environment leads to considerations about the contributions of each to ASD's onset and severity. The study of the interaction between biology and the environment, known as epigenetics, is a field of intensive research. Such an understanding is entirely practical because if biology is destiny and ASD is fully a genetic phenomenon, then the only solution is gene therapy, an active branch of medicine still in its early stages. If, on the other hand, the environment plays the decisive role in ASD's onset and severity, then it becomes imperative to ensure the best upbringing, care, and education of children worldwide.

As noted earlier, the more genes two people share, the greater the number of attributes they share. Suppose that a boy named Tom has ASD. Taking the direct relationship between the number of genes and the number of traits shared as a guide, ASD is likeliest to beset Tom's closest relatives. Parents and ordinary siblings are at greatest risk because, on average, Tom will share half his genes with each parent and each sibling. But circumstances change if Tom has an identical twin because identical twins, being genetic equivalents, are the same genotype and so share the same genes. Keep in mind that the existence of a fraternal twin will not be as helpful because fraternal twins share half their genes even though they happen to have been born at the same time. The key point is that if ASD is under genetic control and if Tom has an identical twin, then that twin should also have ASD.

Research on identical twins demonstrates that an identical twin is ten times more likely to have ASD if his or her genetic equivalent has it than the fraternal twin of someone with ASD. This result is significant because of the expectation that a fraternal twin should have ASD if the other twin has the disorder and environmental factors are identical given that fraternal twins share the same womb. Even immediately after birth, the two should thrive or flounder in the same environment because hospital conditions should be uniform. But the greater occurrence of ASD between identical twins than between fraternal twin is strong evidence that genes must be more important than the environment, so that biology must largely set the conditions for ASD's onset and severity. Keep in mind, however, that not every identical twin of a person with ASD has ASD, a discrepancy that implies some role for the environment.

The results of identical twin studies banish the prospect of ending ASD through superior social engineering. The best parenting, upbringing, care, and education may not be enough to overcome biology. This reality does not necessarily lead to pessimism; in a sense this news is encouraging as it absolves parents from guilt that their parenting made a child autistic. The refrigerator mom thesis being wrong, the medical community strives to extend the greatest compassion and empathy to parents.

The environmental argument may be tested another way. If familial ties are unimportant, other factors should come to the fore. For instance, ASD might cluster by neighborhoods, which tend to be uniform in terms of incomes and even mindsets. But this expectation, at least in economic terms, cannot be true because, as chapter 2 stated, Leo Kanner and Hans Asperger mostly treated children from affluent families whereas Loretta Bender treated the poor. This diversity of economic circumstances must weaken the claim that such factors are very relevant to ASD's onset and severity.

These factors being under consideration, it is unsurprising that interest in family ties remains robust and that researchers are intent on tracing ASD in families in the way that the agronomist traces patterns of inheritance in corn plants that display curious traits. As noted elsewhere, such research establishes that families with an ASD member are at risk that another family member will have ASD. Furthermore, the link is stronger in nuclear families than in extended families because nuclear families have closely related kin like mothers and sons, whereas extended families have less closely related members like cousins, uncles, aunts, nieces, and nephews.

Perhaps the most interesting facet of this research, as noted elsewhere, is the conclusion that inheritance patterns must be more complex than Mendel had thought. He had experimented with pea plants, which display simple patterns of inheritance. He accounted for this simplicity by assuming that each trait is under the control of a single version of a gene and that these versions come in pairs. That is, he postulated a one-to-one relationship between a version of a gene and a trait such that height in a pea plant, for example, is under the control of a single gene variant. But this linear thinking has ceded ground to the realization that, at least in humans, most traits depend on interactions among many genes to express an aspect of the phenotype. This insight is gratifying because it accounts for marked variations in ASD's severity. Were ASD under the control of a single gene, a person would either have it or not without any gradation in signs and symptoms. But this is untrue because ASD presents as severe in someone with many harmful genes, whereas a person who presents mild signs and symptoms has fewer faulty genes. In the language of science, ASD must be a multi-genetic trait. This result is unsurprising given that lots of human traits are under multi-genetic control. A glimpse at the people on any street corner reveals a range of heights, skin colors, intelligences, and innumerable other attributes.

Even so, genes cannot be the whole story. Consider two identical twins and suppose that one eats lean meats, chicken, fish, and plenty of fresh fruits and vegetables, whereas the other consumes nothing but cupcakes. Diet is an environmental factor, and the responsible physician must favor a nutritious, balanced diet over junk foods.

There is yet another way to gauge the contributions of biology and the environment to ASD's onset and severity. Suppose two parents have a single biological child named Randall and a single adopted child named Richard. Gender cannot be a factor because Randall and Richard are both boys. Now suppose that one parent has ASD. If it is under genetic control, Randall should be more likely to have ASD than Richard if neither of Richard's biological parents has ASD. If, however, the environment is the key factor, Randall and Richard should be at equal risk of having ASD because both grow up in an environment with one parent who has ASD. The fact that the adult with ASD is the biological parent of Randall whereas he or she is merely the adoptive parent of Richard should make no difference, but research debunks this line of reasoning, demonstrating instead that Randall is at greater risk than Richard of having ASD.

None of the foregoing diminishes the environment's importance or discounts that the interaction between biology and environment modifies ASD's severity. In other words, biology determines who has ASD whereas the environment helps set its magnitude such that a healthful environment may diminish signs and symptoms whereas a detrimental one may worsen them.

CONCLUSION

This chapter has linked the contributions of biology and the environment to ASD's onset and severity. A study of biology must include genetics because genes establish the species' genotypes, an insight that shapes knowledge about ASD because ASD arises from defects to a genotype. Multiple studies appear to confirm that genes more than the environment control ASD's onset and severity. But these circumstances are not grounds for despair because all children deserve the best upbringing, nurturing, nutrition, education, prospects for earning a living wage, medical care, and quality of life, without which no one can hope to reach his or her potential. In a fundamental way, the nature versus nurture debate does not alter the reality of ASD. Whatever the causes and risk factors, its signs and symptoms must be recognized so that medical practitioners may move toward treatment and management. Chapter 4 focuses on these signs and symptoms, and chapter 5 examines the treatment and management options that follow diagnosis.

4

Signs and Symptoms

Regardless of its causes and risk factors, autism spectrum disorder (ASD) is identified at least partly by its signs and symptoms. Casual use of language might combine these terms, but this chapter differentiates sign from symptom. A sign refers to anything that a physician might notice in a patient, whereas a symptom is something that the patient notices without the intervention of a medical practitioner. This distinction between the two terms does not mean that the two never overlap. Consider a man with arthritic knees. Discomfort may cause him to limp, a condition that cannot escape his notice such that it must be a symptom. In visiting the doctor to discuss the matter, he may sit in a chair while awaiting her. The position stiffens his knees, a condition that worsens his arthritis so that when he stands and steps forward to greet the doctor upon her arrival, she cannot fail to notice the limp. What was a symptom to him is now a sign to her.

Although it is not difficult to describe the signs and symptoms of ASD, their causes are less easily pinpointed. Researchers still have much work to do to detail them. Sometimes the most a researcher can do is to suggest that some region of the brain must not function as it should. At the core, ASD is a neurological condition that necessarily focuses attention on the brain and the rest of the central nervous system (CNS). The genes inherited at conception guide CNS development, strongly suggesting that ASD's signs and symptoms, present in some form very early in life, are under genetic control.

SIGNS AND SYMPTOMS ON THE SPECTRUM

Previous chapters emphasize that ASD is not a binary condition that someone has or does not have in the way that a standard light fixture is either on or off. Rather ASD exhibits a vast range, or spectrum, of characteristics. It may be compared to a dimmer light that has a broad range of luminosities, so that when it is on low it may glow faintly and at the other extreme it may emit bright light. Between these poles is a large range of luminosities.

Because of its variations, ASD is a continuum of signs and symptoms that themselves can vary markedly in severity. A person with ASD may have mild signs and symptoms and the ability to mask them such that social situations, work, errands, theater attendance, and other settings betray no apparent discomfort in his or her behavior. On the other hand, signs and symptoms may be so severe that the sufferer cannot function in society, at least not independently, and so must depend on others or government for care.

This section cannot hope to cover all bases, though an example might move us in the right direction. It has long been known that ASD may cause a range of cognitive signs and symptoms. Recall from chapter 2, for example, that Austrian pediatrician Hans Asperger treated children who displayed no cognitive difficulties. Instead he witnessed richness and range of language as they described their passions. This richness demonstrated cognitive gifts rather than deficits.

Yet it is equally clear that many people with ASD experience more difficulties. Some sufferers exhibit marked cognitive deficits. Researchers have tried to quantify these deficits by measuring a person's intelligence quotient (IQ), which purports to derive from a fraction with mental age in the numerator and chronological age in the denominator. The more gifted the person the higher should be mental age relative to chronological age, enlarging the quotient. At the other extreme, deficits might lower mental age below chronological age, shrinking the quotient. A score of 100 (really 1.00), signifying that mental and chronological ages are equal, is considered average. Some people with ASD score below 70, which is considered mentally deficient, and suffer marked cognitive impairment.

Even so, caution is warranted. Researchers derive IQ from a person's performance on a test. An onlooker might wonder about the validity of extrapolating performance on a single test or even a series of tests to generalize about someone's entire set of cognitive abilities. Critics of IQ tests have included the late Harvard University evolutionary biologist and geologist Stephen Jay Gould, whose book *The Mismeasure of Man* (1996) provides a good introduction to the topic and related errors.

SOCIAL DEFICITS AS SIGNS AND SYMPTOMS

Because most humans are intensely gregarious, social deficits were among the first signs and symptoms to identify ASD. Asperger, whose pioneering work in the 1930s and 1940s at least partly shaped the future of ASD research and treatment, was among the first to note its social deficiencies. These problems are numerous and sometimes striking because they set the person with ASD apart from those who perceive themselves as normal. Here the term "normal," sometimes labeled neurotypical in the scientific and medical literature, just means a person whose behavior lies within the largest part of the bell curve. The abnormal person, if such language must be used, is just an outlier on the bell curve with no value judgment implied.

Among ASD's social deficits is difficulty decoding others' intentions. The ability to perceive intentions is fundamental to any social interaction, and people routinely signal their intentions in a variety of ways. Verbal cues are sometimes easy to understand, but nonverbal cues, often tethered to body language and facial expression, often elude a person with ASD such that he or she is either unsure of another's intentions or mistakes them for something else. Such mistakes cause misunderstandings even though a person with ASD strives to understand intentions and motivations. The failure to do so erroneously marks him or her as inattentive or dull witted. The problem is worse because he or she may be unaware of being judged so harshly. In ASD's worst cases, a person may be unable to interact with others at even the most superficial level. Even family and friends may be able to form only tenuous bonds with him or her. These complications fall under nonprofit advocacy group Autism Speaks' definition of ASD. Its PDF "About Autism" summarizes ASD's social deficits.

Part of the problem, the Indiana Resource Center for Autism at Indiana University in Bloomington notes, stems from a person with ASD's difficulty communicating with others, a topic that receives more attention in the next section. Here it suffices to note that a host of troubles may weaken these attempts, even in mild cases of ASD. Difficulty initiating and maintaining eye contact is well known. It is not a sign of disrespect but is so ingrained as to be more reflex than conscious decision, an aversion detailed by the charitable organization Staffordshire Adults Autistic Society in Newcastle, England. Absent eye contact, a person with ASD can neither perceive another's intentions and motivations nor communicate his own intentions directly and efficiently. The other conversant, perceiving the person's difficulties, is likely to notice inadequate eye contact rather than his or her words. In this way and without malicious intent, a person with ASD has made an unsettling impression on the listener, derailing the conversation. With ineffective or transitory eye contact, a person with ASD may display awkward gestures and body language that further muddy the message. Confusion rather than communication results. In the worst instances, a person with ASD looks at a distant object rather than his or her conversant.

Even under the best circumstances, communication is ineffective in a person with ASD who is unmotivated to engage another, a problem examined in the National Public Radio January 2009 program "Teaching Kids with Autism the Art of Conversation." People without ASD tend to underestimate the exertion necessary to engage in conversation. A person with ASD toils under this constraint even as he tries to disguise his distress. Rather than engage the listener, he may withdraw from lack of energy to sustain a conversation, fearing that it might last too long or require too much attentiveness. Even a few minutes of banter may exhaust him when the other is just hitting her stride and is ready to discuss substantive matters. By then he may have withdrawn from the conversation and so has missed its most consequential parts. This withdrawal is marked in ASD's severe cases, such that he seems to inhabit his own world.

Erratic and incomplete social engagement has another component in that a person with ASD may display antisocial behaviors (Rutter, Giller, and Hagell 1998). In this context, a person with ASD does not seek attention through aberrant behaviors because they function as a coping mechanism to release tension even though they discomfort others. Unfortunately, the public seldom perceives the primacy of releasing tension, only the behavior's jarring nature. Because tension must be released, a person with ASD may continue to act out even as others try to calm him. Such interventions further distress the public. Discomfort mounts the longer and more ineffective are attempts to restore calm. Antisocial behaviors may stem from what may be termed hyper vigilance against perceived threats.

Such behaviors, labeled tantrums, begin early in life and are inevitable. Such instances are not mysterious given that children have not developed mechanisms to cope effectively with negative stimuli. Children with ASD are no different, but their tantrums may be especially frequent, violent, persistent, and difficult to control or minimize. Such problems may fray the nerves of even the calmest parents. Hard data do not exist to tabulate the frequency of these tantrums, though Shannon (2011) notes their pervasiveness.

Some children with ASD improve as they mature. They have not outgrown their ASD even when signs and symptoms become less alarming. Even under the best circumstances, however, an adult with ASD may lose his temper. At one extreme, he may become aggressive when excited or fearful. Again, coping mechanisms become inadequate. Aggression may take several forms including an attempt to inflict physical harm. This behavior is evident in our closest kin, the chimpanzee and gorilla, but is usually for show, especially in the gorilla.

At other times aggression may be passive and include a refusal to comply with ordinary, reasonable requests or directives. Such resistance may cause anguish at work for both employer and employee because an employer has the right to direct employees' actions toward profitability and will perceive any noncompliance as defiance. Discipline may lead to termination. Such dynamics explain why adults with ASD may have gaps in their employment or difficulty holding a job very long, problems that receive commentary in Virginia Commonwealth University Autism Resource Center's "Employment and Adults with Autism Spectrum Disorders: Challenges and Strategies for Success." First person accounts of these difficulties populate the Internet. Episodic employment may cause adults with ASD to struggle against being perceived as jobs jumpers.

LANGUAGE AND COMMUNICATION DEFICITS

Related to social deficits are language and communication problems, whose difficulties are seldom overstated because language is basic to humans. Indeed, the acquisition of language seems to be a hallmark of humanity. It appears that no other species has developed speech, reading, and writing. Given language's prominence, anyone deficient in communication risks separation from the world of ideas and interactions.

In ASD, language deficits emerge early in life, a fact documented by many agencies including the U.S. National Library of Medicine's National Center for Biotechnology Information in Bethesda, Maryland. Infancy is devoid of language even though it seems clear that babies can and do communicate with their parents in a variety of verbal and nonverbal ways. After infancy, however, children typically acquire language at an astonishing rate. But here children with ASD falter so that parents know almost immediately that their child is lagging in language. In other cases, a child with ASD may develop some language at the outset only to regress around age two such that this age marks a milestone in ASD's detection because worried parents rush their child to the pediatrician before the next scheduled visit.

Whatever the rate of language acquisition, the amount varies. Some children with ASD develop language with limited vocabulary. Silence results when the language landscape is barren. Silence alarms parents, who fear their child is deaf. An ASD diagnosis brings relief that he or she can hear but also fear of a condition they had not suspected. The earliest medical interventions hold the greatest potential for improvement.

Babies with ASD may be unusually quiet. Attentive parents may be attuned to several early problems including the absence of babbling. A baby with ASD may be notably irritable and difficult to console when upset, problems that foreshadow the tantrums that mar childhood. Such babies may make poor eye contact, a trait that often persists throughout life. Babies with ASD, absorbed in their own world, may be quiet because they want to interact with objects rather than people. In extreme cases, babies with ASD may not respond to parents' voices. Such behavior again brings on the crisis that leads to a diagnosis of ASD rather than deafness.

Whatever these deficits, parents soon realize that their child's poor acquisition of language and communication takes many forms. Children with ASD who speak infrequently if at all develop other capacities. For example, an ASD child who wants a toy may point rather than ask for it. In other instances, children with ASD may act as if alone even in public or at school, ignoring potential playmates and failing to reciprocate their attention. Whereas other children engross themselves in the activities of others, an ASD child may manipulate an object alone for long periods. In such instances the quiet autistic baby develops into a child whose silence draws attention from teachers, who may alert parents of his or her need for medical attention. An ASD child's silence is directed not just at teachers but also at schoolmates. A child with ASD who seldom talks to peers often matures into an adult who has trouble interacting with colleagues at work.

Problems with language and communication may affect other capacities. The most basic may stem from ASD people's literal interpretation of language, a fact documented and summarized in PsychologyToday.com's "People with Autism Spectrum Disorder Take Things Literally." This concern has nothing to do with bible literalism; rather the effects touch many aspects of life. For example, a person with ASD may enjoy the keyboard works of eighteenth century German composer Johann Sebastian Bach but may believe that because Bach composed them for the harpsichord they may not be performed on the piano. This literal fidelity to the harpsichord may prevent enjoyment of pianistic interpretations. Such thoughts may seem inconsequential, but literalness can be an impediment, as when a job description is interpreted in such a narrow way that the applicant fails to understand that a desk job nonetheless requires interaction with people. Human resources seldom bothers to state the obvious so that the burden always falls on the applicant.

Existence within narrow literal parameters may impede basic reasoning by diminishing the capacity to make an inference, a type of conclusion drawn from a statement. For example, the statement that Earth is a planet and so orbits the Sun should prompt the inference that all the other planets in our solar system must also orbit the Sun. Yet a literal preoccupation with Earth may impede a person with ASD from considering the movements of the other planets. Such literalness hinders learning.

Language deficits, evident early, hinder the acquisition of words and are notable in children with ASD who struggle to memorize their meaning. Sometimes they acquire nouns more readily than other parts of language, but even then they tend to forget nouns so that learning always seems to mean relearning; meanwhile neurotypical children surge ahead by retaining nouns and other parts of speech in their memory. When impairment is severe enough, children with ASD cannot recall the names of relatives and other close companions. Some people with ASD have almost no capacity for language. They may emit occasional sounds, but these vocalizations appear to lack meaning. At other times barren language leads to silence.

These deficits point to cognitive impairments that result in low IQs and the stigma of mental retardation. This chapter notes the problem of reification. Nonetheless, IQ seems to provide some mechanism for ranking the severity of mental retardation. Social scientists and medical practitioners tend to divide it into three categories. The least severe cases have an IQ between roughly 50 and 70. Such individuals are thought to be mildly retarded. Moderate retardation is between roughly 30 and 50. The most severe cases dip below 30.

The most severe instances are sometimes labeled profound mental retardation. In these cases, the prospects for independent living are improbable if not impossible. Through careful instruction such a person may learn the rudiments of self-care and may vocalize sounds in hopes of eliciting a caregiver's attention. Often, he or she progresses no further, retaining the characteristics of a preliterate child throughout life. Such a person worries family and friends as they struggle to help him or her cope with the rudiments of existence, evoking seventeenth century English philosopher and political writer Thomas Hobbes' description of life, in its natural state, as "solitary, poor, nasty, brutish, and short."

Nonetheless, language and communication problems are not always a sure guide to ASD's presence and severity because some children with ASD display no such deficits, as Hans Asperger noted in the 1930s and 1940s. Recall that he studied children who displayed social deficits but whose language was adequate and sometimes even exceptional. He encountered children who relished the opportunity to discuss their interests in such detail that Asperger likened them to "little professors." Rather than deficient, these children had a superabundance of language. Moreover, language deficits are not unique to ASD. Several types of brain damage also impair language. Even some healthy, neurotypical people never master the ability to write even three consecutive sentences, the first logically necessitating the second, and the second in turn leading inexorably to the third. These facts demonstrate that language and communication deficiencies by themselves do not justify an ASD diagnosis.

BEHAVIORAL DEFICITS

Socialization, language, and other aspects of communication are only part of ASD's story. Behavioral deficits are also signs and symptoms of ASD, as is evident from earlier coverage of antisocial outbursts and inappropriate displays of anger. Of course, anyone can become angry during a tumultuous experience, but society expects him or her to mask or suppress this anger or otherwise channel it in a benign direction. Such mastery of emotions can be difficult for people with ASD who erupt in anger in the way that an overinflated tire may rupture without warning. This release can be sudden and volatile, discomforting onlookers. Some people without ASD are subject to such outbursts. Violent criminals end up in prison for this reason. Nonetheless, these episodes may be particularly difficult for people with ASD to control. Tempestuous outbursts, like antisocial behaviors in general, may derive from the hyper vigilance mentioned earlier.

These outbursts betray the deeper problem of impulse control, a well-established ASD feature. Of course, impulses are an important component of life. In some ways, sex can be an impulse when the attraction between two people is elemental. Yet existence within society requires some sublimation of impulses. No man, for example, can have sex with every woman he sees. Such behavior would disrupt society in serious and dangerous ways. But a person with ASD's trouble suppressing impulses prevents him or her from obtaining a greater reward later so that the concept of delayed gratification may be foreign to him or her. Again, the ability to delay gratification is not unique to people with ASD. Criminals and those who amass debts, especially because of impulsive purchasing habits, often cannot or will not delay their desire to have or do sometime at the spur of the moment.

Some people with ASD display other contrary behaviors including resistance to authority, a trait known as Pathological Demand Avoidance. This resistance may not arise from outright defiance, but the authority tends to interpret resistance as defiance and to brand the person with ASD as subversive. Exchanges between a person with ASD and a teacher or police officer may become tense even when inconsequential matters are under consideration. The causes of resistance to authority are difficult to pinpoint, though again some criminals must have this trait even when they do not have ASD. ASD people's resistance to authority probably differs from criminal tendencies in this direction.

Such behavioral deficits may interfere with a capacity for sustained activity, manifesting, for example, as difficulty concentrating. Here ASD overlaps with various hyperactivity and inattention deficits and with other maladies like schizophrenia, accounting for the fact that some people with ASD do not excel in schoolwork. People like American livestock expert

Temple Grandin, who has ASD and was mentioned in chapters 2 and 3 and who has a PhD from a distinguished land grant university, are notable because they are the exception rather than the rule. Inattentiveness has a corollary in difficulty completing tasks. Again, Grandin is noteworthy for completing all coursework and the dissertation for her PhD.

Inattentiveness spills over into other aspects of a person with ASD's life. Inattentiveness coupled with hyperactivity may delay him or her from settling into a routine because disruption causes discomfort, a facet of ASD seemingly at odds with a preference for repetition and sameness. Employers may be uneasy with such employees in the conviction that they adapt poorly to new directives and abrupt changes in the workplace. The preference for repetition is evident in people with ASD who spend long intervals listening to the same piece of music many times. Odd as it may seem, such behavior comforts those with ASD, who equate change with disruption. In these cases, change presages disorder and disorientation. The tension between aversion of routine and preference for repetition underscores the reality that ASD affects different people in different ways.

Preference for routine and repetition narrows the range of activities and interests. Such preoccupation can yield fruit. It is hard, for example, to imagine that luminaries like English polymath Isaac Newton or German physicist and Nobel laureate Albert Einstein could have reached the apex of intellectual achievement without a single-minded devotion to science. But in people with ASD such devotion can become obsessive. Those absorbed in routine and repetition tend to become rigid. In the worst cases repetition includes a range of alarming behaviors like excessive rocking, arm waving, hand and finger movements, rigid postures, and injuries when a person with ASD bangs his head, bites himself, scratches himself inordinately, or hits himself with objects.

The impulse toward self-injury afflicts people with severe ASD, who may break bones and teeth, detach the retinas by jabbing fingers into their eyes, and cause concussions, requiring medical intervention. Even medical efforts may not prevent such people from killing themselves. The Children's Hospital of Philadelphia rates these behaviors as uncommon but notable in cognitively impaired people with ASD. The next section examines these behaviors in light of ASD tactile abnormalities.

Institutions cope with these behaviors as best they can, putting severely ASD people in helmets, knee pads, and arm and leg splits. Sometimes restraints are necessary. The medical community has labeled such violence self-injurious behaviors (SIB), which, like language and communication problems, do not alone necessitate a diagnosis of ASD, whose range of signs and symptoms require multiple lines of evidence to confirm it. ASD's complexities contribute to the fact that some people with ASD receive inaccurate diagnoses or escape detection until adulthood.

SENSORY ABNORMALITIES

As in many other ASD signs and symptoms, sensory problems may be difficult to categorize because of their different effects on different people. Empiricism and common sense hold that humans derive information through the senses, a perspective that seems to contradict the way people learn mathematics. Defects in sensory perceptions disadvantage people with ASD in their efforts to cope with daily life. Signs and symptoms range from insensitivity to sensory stimuli to hypersensitivity. Some people with ASD may be virtually unable to detect odors, hear sounds distinctly, or feel their surroundings through touch. Others are hypersensitive to stimuli. It is interesting to note the story about one esteemed conductor suspected of being autistic who cautioned women in the audience not to open or close their purses during a performance because the accumulation of these sounds impaired his ability to conduct the orchestra.

Other hypersensitive autistics are inordinately sensitive to light, prompting them to turn off all lights in the evening. Even winter's dreariness seldom coaxes them to turn on a light at home or the office during the day. Even light from a television may cause discomfort. Another interesting anecdote holds that a prominent and possibly autistic philosopher of the early twentieth century never booked any hotel room unless he could be assured that no light penetrated the window drapes at night. He apparently inspected these rooms with great care to ensure that they met his specifications before he would admit his luggage.

SLEEP DISORDERS

Humans have long intuited the importance of sleep. Recent research illuminates just how essential it is. We now know that adequate sleep is necessary to form long term memories. Without such rest, the brain cannot encode significant events in the memory, and a person with memory deficits is not him or herself in significant ways. Someone who can no longer recall grandchildren's names, for example, has lost an important part of his or her identity.

The problems with sleep irregularities in people with ASD include disruption of the circadian rhythm. Basic to our biology, the circadian rhythm is an internal clock that tells us when to sleep and when to be awake. This system may seem so mundane as to be trivial, but such a perspective is untrue because our circadian rhythm conditions us to be active during the day and sleepy at night, the reverse of the pattern for many other mammals. This peculiarity must have long been vital to our success as a species because, alert during the day, hunter gatherers could track, kill, and eat other mammals at exactly the time when they were sluggish and less able to evade humans. Disruption of the circadian rhythm thus runs counter to our evolutionary history.

Yet this disruption plagues some people with ASD. The problem is rooted in biology because the brain regulates the production of several chemicals that govern wakefulness or sleepiness. Two chemicals deserve particular attention. The first, gamma aminobutyric acid (GABA), is a neurotransmitter originating in the hypothalamus, an ancient region of the brain that facilitates communication between the central nervous system (CNS) and the endocrine system. ASD, being a neurological condition, necessarily affects the CNS.

Returning to the circadian rhythm, GABA tells the body when to awaken. Without it no one can hope to be alert enough to conquer each day's demands. When GABA is deficient, people with ASD feel sluggish throughout the day. Such impairment disrupts normal activities like work and errands. These people are not lazy even though an employer may question their work ethic. Such problems mar some people with ASD's work histories.

Research and the media have raised the profile of the second chemical, melatonin. The pineal gland regulates its production, an action that is not just biological because the gland responds to light to regulate the amount of melatonin in the body. When light is abundant in daytime, the pineal gland suppresses melatonin production to heighten wakefulness. In light's absence during night, the pineal gland produces melatonin to relax the body in preparation for sleep. Without this fine tuning, a person cannot sleep when environmental cues favor restfulness, disrupting the circadian rhythm.

This focus on the CNS and on chemicals in the brain has other troubling aspects. Aside from the hypothalamus, another part of the brain, the brainstem, is also central to the regulation of sleep. The fact that many animal species have a brainstem implies that it is among the oldest, if not the oldest, regions of the brain. Its importance to several biological processes can scarcely be overstated because the brainstem acts in many ways as the brain's command and control center, regulating the flow of chemicals between the brain and the rest of the body. These chemicals are really information, meaning that the brainstem supplies the biochemical information necessary for the rest of the body to function. One measure of the brainstem's importance lies in its regulation of breathing, heart rate, swallowing, blood pressure, consciousness, and, crucially for our purposes, sleepiness.

The brainstem does not always function optimally in people with ASD so that as many as 83 percent of children with ASD suffer from insomnia, their most common physical complaint. Anyone who has endured an occasional restless night can guess how debilitating insomnia must be and how much these children must suffer. Note that insomnia is not just an episodic complaint. By its nature insomnia is a habitual problem that afflicts people night after night. Chronic sleeplessness worsens daytime. Afflicted children have difficulty concentrating in school, a circumstance that at least partly explains why some children with ASD perform poorly in their studies. Afflicted adults struggle to remain alert at work and to summon the energy for the errands and chores of daily existence. As with disruptions to the circadian rhythm, insomnia contributes to the poor work histories of some adults with ASD.

ASD sleep disturbances may take other forms. Under the heading of primary sleep disorders are uncontrolled movements of the arms and legs, generally known as periodic limb movement. When the condition troubles just the legs, it is usually known as restless leg syndrome. A neurotypical person may experience these problems, but they are more pervasive and troublesome among people with ASD. These involuntary movements may be so sudden and violent that a physician may suspect epilepsy rather than ASD, an unsurprising situation given that some epileptics have ASD too because both are neurological afflictions. These problems worsen insomnia because a sufferer may retire to bed in hopes of sleeping only to have these movements keep him or her awake. Primary sleep disorders thus complicate insomnia by erecting additional barriers to the body's attempts to sleep. Several areas of the brain, notably the motor cortex, control the limbs such that its defects must at least partly account for the severity of periodic limb movement and restless leg syndrome.

Other conditions may be present, including disruption of rapid eye movement (REM) during sleep. Medical practitioners understand that the eyeballs move quickly when a person dreams and that REM is necessary for a person to dream. Dreaming may seem inconsequential at least partly because dreams often seem disordered and difficult to interpret. But studies demonstrate that anyone deprived of REM, and thus of dreaming, for several nights will suffer psychosis even if the duration of sleep is adequate. Such REM disturbances thus predispose people with ASD to mental problems. The relationship between REM and ASD requires more research to understand why people with ASD are subject to REM disturbances. The regions of the brain known as the pons and medulla play a large role in controlling REM so that their defects must disrupt REM as well as heighten ASD's severity.

Another ASD problem are night terrors in both children and adults. Note that night terrors are not nightmares, which are a type of frightful dream. But a night terror is no dream because it does not seem to occur during REM as nightmares do. Rather it originates during the deepest moments of sleep, when a person should be most relaxed. Instead of relaxation, a night terror awakens a person suddenly and in great fear. He or she may emerge from a night terror with a shirt wet from sweat and may even be sweating upon arousal. Such terrors delay or prevent the sufferer from returning to sleep. During deep sleep, the brain should be most at rest, but when parts of it experience unusual activity, night terrors result. Their causes include insufficient sleep in previous nights, a bladder that is too full, fever, emotional upheaval, noise, light, and medications that alter the CNS. In the last case a pharmacist or doctor should alert a person with ASD about this side effect.

Alternatively, people with ASD may experience disturbances that awaken them suddenly and early in the morning. Despite their best efforts, sleep does not return so that they must either lie awake or begin the day. Other abnormalities include sleepwalking, a condition that occurs without any conscious control of the body. Because the hypothalamus regulates sleepiness and wakefulness, its defects likely cause some episodes of early awakening in people with ASD.

Another malady is bruxism, the grinding and clenching of teeth during sleep. The condition tends to persist violently in people with ASD. Undetected, bruxism damages teeth. In serious cases teeth are so broken or worn that extraction is necessary. Once aware of the problem, sufferers may wear a mouth guard for protection. A mouth guard often has a short lifespan because bruxism causes a person to chew through it. Stress, anxiety, sleep apnea, or missing or misaligned teeth can cause bruxism. Sleep apnea interrupts breathing during sleep, even to the point of stopping breathing momentarily, and is often severe in people with ASD. Although sleep apnea appears to correlate with obesity, this link is not absolute in people with ASD because it is also prevalent among lean and fit people with ASD who should not ordinarily be at risk. All the above causes may not operate in any one person with ASD.

POTENTIAL UNDERLYING CAUSES OF ASD'S SIGNS AND SYMPTOMS

Earlier parts of this chapter note several likely causes of one or more ASD signs or symptoms. This section focuses on other probable causes (Shannon 2011; Hollander, Kolevson, and Coyle 2011). Beginning with social deficiencies as signs and symptoms, research points to several causes, including the fact that people with ASD perceive others differently than do neurotypical people. These perceptions may derive from the senses so that insensitivity or hypersensitivity to external stimuli may cause people with ASD to misinterpret intentions. A person with ASD whose hearing is especially acute may perceive every encounter as a threat because of his or her tendency to interpret others' matter of fact comments as menacing. Another avenue of research in social deficits focuses on difficulties in making and sustaining eye contact, possibly caused to some extent by some fundamental discomfort or perhaps hypersensitivity around others, discomfort usually absent in neurotypical people. In a sense, the person with ASD, without making a conscious decision, has become hypervigilant such that anyone anywhere within the field of vision may trigger the sensation of being under assault when no real threat exists.

Social deficits overlap with language and communication problems, including disengagement or withdrawal from conversations, possibly due to inadequate motivation to sustain an encounter, a phenomenon mentioned earlier. This apparent lack of motivation, difficult to explain, aligns ASD with schizophrenia such that a cause or group of causes may explain poor motivation in both. This approach may hamper rather than enhance understanding. Consider the fact that smoking causes some types of cancer. Now elevate this cause and effect relationship to the level of generalization by trying to find a single cause or group of causes of all types of cancer. Such a goal may be achieved in the future, but today it appears to be wishful thinking. Moreover, scientists and doctors may be unable to declare smoking as the universal cause because even though it is responsible for some cancers, it cannot be responsible for all. Research documents cases in which both mother and daughter contract breast cancer although neither smoked a cigarette or even inhaled second hand smoke. Perhaps the decisive fact is that people in the Old World succumbed to various types of cancer before the sixteenth century and so before anyone besides the Amerindians had ever seen a tobacco plant. In other words, even though research will likely proceed against ASD and schizophrenia, no one should expect the discovery of some factor that causes both. In a larger sense, language deficits arise in the brain, but the specific region or regions are difficult to pinpoint because of the generalized character of language comprehension and speech. At a minimum, the frontal, temporal, occipital, and parietal lobes as well as the cerebellum control aspects of language acquisition and manipulation. The causes of language and communication difficulties must lie somewhere in one or more of these regions. Specificity awaits future research.

Earlier commentary noted behaviors that range from repetition and sameness to variable activities because of aversion to routine. These opposites suggest that different causes must be at work. Whenever gradations in behaviors occupy the region between opposites, a continuum results to reinforce ASD's range of signs and symptoms. This circumstance corroborates the knowledge that ASD is no binary condition. Repetitive behaviors originate in the cerebellum so that it must determine their presence or absence. Repetitiveness is thought to preoccupy a person with ASD, thereby diminishing anxiety or other responses to stress. If this rationale is correct, repetitiveness must have roots in our evolution as a mechanism that natural selection favored because it reduces anxiety. Retaining a focus on the brain, sensory problems must originate in the parietal lobe, which receives and interprets stimuli.

As valuable as may be general discussions of potential causes of ASD's signs and symptoms, biological factors locate these causes in the genes, an unsurprising progression given that ASD is a neurological condition present at life's earliest stages. This conviction does not suppose that ASD is full-fledged at conception because the CNS cannot be present then. In other words, ASD is like all biological processes in being a development rather than a sudden manifestation. Chapter 3 accentuated the role of genes in determining ASD's onset and severity, leading us to renew this approach here. Genetic factors are evident from several studies. All cannot receive treatment here except to note that the National Institutes of Health (NIH) in Bethesda, Maryland, regularly publishes authoritative treatments of ASD (National Institutes of Health 2005; National Institutes of Health 2008).

A caveat is in order. This book treats ASD as a malady and its signs and symptoms as evidence that this malady afflicts some people. In this spirit the attempt is made to tease apart the causes of both ASD and its signs and symptoms, if these factors exist in a way that allows more or less independent coverage. Such partitioning is difficult to achieve because it is sometimes possible to cite a factor or group of factors as cause of both malady and its signs and symptoms. For example, and to revive an example from chapter 3, yellow fever virus necessarily causes the tropical disease yellow fever. At the same time, a person infected by the virus develops a horrible fever accompanied by other dire signs and symptoms. In other words, yellow fever virus may logically be inferred as cause of both yellow fever and its signs and symptoms. This connection between affliction and its signs and symptoms must be part of ASD too, so that causes are difficult to partition cleanly between ASD as a reality and ASD as the sum of all its signs and symptoms.

Regarding the foregoing, scientists and physicians acknowledge that they do not precisely know the causes of ASD and its signs and symptoms. Nonetheless, up to 12 genes, not all on a single chromosome, are implicated as possible triggers of ASD's signs and symptoms. Attention focuses on chromosome 2 (remember that a person has 23 pairs or 46 chromosomes), which appears to have genes whose poor functioning may impair the formation and action of the brainstem and cerebellum. Recall that inadequate functioning of the brainstem likely disturbs sleep and that improper activity in the cerebellum may diminish language proficiency. Chromosome 17 appears to have faulty genes that may cause or amplify mental retardation in people with ASD.

This inquiry into the genetic causes of ASD's signs and symptoms receives reinforcement from Sabat (2007), which links certain ASD signs and symptoms to mutations in at least 100 genes, not all on a single chromosome and most if not all acting in concert with other genes. Scientists and physicians hope to identify these genes and understand how their improper functioning may cause some of ASD's signs and symptoms. Because ASD is, at its core, a neurological condition, researchers, after identifying these genes, must describe their biochemical pathways to illuminate how their mutations hamper the brain and the rest of the CNS. Physicians at the National Institute of Mental Health (NIMH) believe that the action of these genes, once understood, may help explain signs and symptoms in as many as 90 percent of people with ASD.

ASD's signs and symptoms may be rooted in imperfect connections among the brain's neurons (National Institutes of Health 2009). Attention focuses on chromosome 5, which contains genes CDH 9 and CDH 10, both of which may weaken these connections in people with ASD and so account at least partly for some signs and symptoms. These genes appear to modify the structure and function of proteins, thereby weakening connections among neurons.

Other NIMH studies posit that the inability of at least one gene to code for its companion protein or proteins may play a part in some people with ASDs' social deficits. Repetitive behaviors may also result from this silent gene, which appears to act on the brain's cortex. "Silence" means that the gene does not function, as though it has been deleted. To use an analogy, a person may keep an old bicycle in the garage even though it no longer works. Because the bike no longer serves any purpose, the owner might set it out for the trash collector, in effect deleting it from the garage.

Other signs and symptoms receive attention. A single imperfect gene may lead to the gastrointestinal problems, mentioned in chapter 1, in some people with ASD (Campbell et al. 2009). Recall that genes come in pairs known as alleles. Accordingly, the gene under investigation, MET rs 1858830, is a variant in a specific pair of alleles.

Hyperactivity in some people with ASD may result from the improper functioning of several genes (Anderson 2010). Recall that hyperactivity is likewise a feature of Attention Deficit Hyperactivity Disorder (ADHD), which is a condition separate from ASD. These genes may play a role in signs and symptoms noted earlier, including aggression and disruptive behaviors, accounting for at least some problems that plague children with ASD in school, the home, and elsewhere.

CONCLUSION

ASD has many signs and symptoms varying in severity because, being a continuum, ASD ranges from mild to severe. Much attention focuses on the social deficits that define ASD in the minds of many. Social deficits are troubling on their own, but people with ASD may also have language and communication problems, though people once categorized with Asperger's syndrome often are proficient in language. Behavioral problems are common and can lead to the perception that people with ASD are antisocial. In addition, ASD may have insensitivity or hypersensitivity to sensory stimuli as a sign or symptom. Sleep may suffer such that insomnia is common among people with ASD. Researchers have not pinpointed the causes of every sign and symptom, but attention has focused and is likely to continue to focus on faulty genes. Amelioration of ASD's signs and symptoms is essential to wellbeing. Accordingly, chapter 5 focuses on prompt diagnosis followed by proper treatment and management of signs and symptoms.

REFERENCES

Anderson, Andrea. 2010. "Researchers Probe Genetic Overlap between ADHD, Autism." *Spectrum*, April 22. https://www.spectrumnews.org/news/researchers-probe-genetic-overlap-between-adhd-autism/.

Campbell, D. B., T. M. Buie, H. Winter, M. Bauman, J. S. Sutcliffe, J. M. Perrin, and P. Levitt. 2009. "Distinct Genetic Risk Based on Association of MET in Families with Co-occurring Autism and Gastrointestinal Conditions." *Pediatrics* 123, no. 4: 1255.

Gould, Stephen Jay. 1996. *The Mismeasure of Man.* New York: W. W. Norton.

Hollander, Eric, Alex Kolevson, and Joseph T. Coyle. 2011. *Textbook of Autism Spectrum Disorders.* Washington, DC: American Psychiatric Publishing.

National Institutes of Health. 2005. "Autism and Genes." Bethesda, MD: National Institute of Health. NIH Pub. No. 05–5590. https://files.eric.ed.gov/fulltext/ED485722.pdf.

National Institutes of Health. 2008. "Autism Risk Higher in People with Gene Variant." January 10. https://www.nih.gov/news-events/news-releases/autism-risk-higher-people-gene-variant.

National Institutes of Health. 2009. "Risk of Autism Tied to Genes That Influence Brain Cell Connections." April 28. Press release. https://www.nih.gov/news-events/news-releases/risk-autism-tied-genes-influence-brain-cell-connections.

Rutter, Michael, Henri Giller, and Ann Hagell. 1998. *Antisocial Behavior in Young People: A Major New Review*. Cambridge, UK: Cambridge University Press.

Sebat, J. B. Lakshmi, D. Malhotra, J. E. Troge, C. Lese-Martin, T. Walsh, B. Yamrom, et al. 2007. "Strong Association of De Novo Copy Number Mutations with Autism." *Science*, 316, no. 5823: 445–449.

Shannon, Joyce Brennfleck. 2011. *Autism and Pervasive Developmental Disorders Sourcebook*. 2nd ed. Detroit: Omnigraphics.

5

Diagnosis, Treatment, and Management

Chapter 4 examined the notable symptoms and signs of autism spectrum disorder (ASD), which are the basis for diagnosis. That is, a physician uses these signs and symptoms to diagnose a person as having ASD in the way that a mechanic uses an automobile's observable problems to determine what must be fixed. But diagnosis is just the starting point in that it alone does nothing beyond naming the problem. There is no point, to return to the earlier example, to knowing that a car's tires are excessively worn if neither owner nor mechanic replaces them. The knowledge gained in diagnosis must translate into action to be more than an exercise in manipulating language. In this vein, an ASD diagnosis must lead to a plan of treatment and management, as will be discussed in this chapter. Nowhere does responsible research pretend that a single, foolproof cure for ASD exists. The keys are treatment and management that alleviate symptoms and signs rather than chasing the mirage of a cure that does not now exist. But modern medicine is not defective because every worthwhile endeavor works at the boundary of the unknown in pursuing problems that are now unsolvable.

DIAGNOSIS

The absence of a cure stiffens efforts against ASD. The first step is diagnosis of all ASD cases, no matter how mild. In medicine, diagnosis often requires measurement, a method that cannot surprise anyone who has used a thermometer to quantify a fever's magnitude. This situation applies to ASD, in which researchers have devised tests to gauge its severity as part of diagnosis. These tests evaluate different aspects of a person, central among them being an assessment of cognition as a diagnostic tool.

Measurements of Cognition

Because ASD emerges early in life, the Wechsler intelligence scale for children aims to prompt the earliest ASD diagnosis, an obvious goal given that the earliest diagnosis yields the best prognosis. As the name implies, this test uses a numerical index to quantify ASD's severity just as a thermometer has a number scale to quantify a fever. Analogies along these lines demonstrate that quantification is essential to medicine. Nothing is strange here because the physical sciences like physics and chemistry rely heavily on measurement and quantification.

The Wechsler scale is like an IQ test in attempting to quantify cognition. The defects of such an approach have already been mentioned in previous chapters. The Wechsler scale is thought to allow a medical practitioner to quantify distractibility with a test short enough not to fray a child's nerves given that people with ASD are sometimes easily derailed from completing a task, a phenomenon not unique to ASD. The scale also attempts to quantify the range of a person's language given that cognitive deficits often shrink vocabularies, a point made in the previous chapter. The scale, furthermore, attempts to quantify a person's perceptual acuity. Such attributes cannot be easily quantified even if measurement is truly possible. No single test, not the Wechsler scale or anything else in vogue, provides a complete understanding of ASD. Note that different versions of the test are tailored to children and adults. Hard data do not exist to rank how often the Wechsler scale is used to measure cognition in children and adults, but the U.S. National Library of Medicine at the National Institutes of Health in Bethesda, Maryland, asserts that scientists and medical practitioners use the scale more than any other cognitive test. Regarding an adult, the consensus holds that no test can truly identify ASD in him or her. Chapter 4 elaborates this point and echoes private and public organizations that request more money to fund more research on adults with ASD.

Another quantifier is the differential ability scale, but research casts doubt on its precision. Scores for one individual, both verbal and nonverbal, tend to vary widely even when he or she takes the test repeatedly over a short duration. Moreover, the scale reveals little about an ASD person's social ineptitude because of its underlying premise that strong verbal skills correlate with strong social skills. Even if such correlation is valid, a truism holds that correlation does not prove causation so that even if this scale can identify social deficiencies, it cannot identify their cause or causes. Even people with ASD that are fluent in language may experience profound social deficits. Given these defects, it is natural to wonder how often the scale, for which multiple versions exist, is used on children and adults who possibly have ASD. Another study by the U.S. National Library of Medicine notes that scores from the differential ability scale tend to decline from early childhood to adulthood but does not indicate how often researchers and medical experts use it on children and adults suspected of having ASD. Declining scores imply that the test is used first on children and thereafter repeated into adulthood. Furthermore, the National Library of Medicine states that the scale is only as good as the participants because some children tested at an early age fall through the cracks by age 19 such that they are no longer tested. These people may drop out because diminishing scores cause them to dislike the scale. This information exists within the context that most people dislike tests, whatever their nature, throughout life. This chapter emphasizes that few people have ever liked standardized tests given their use in schools to help decide who merits promotion or a high school diploma.

A third test, the autism spectrum quotient, is a variant of IQ tests. For this reason, proponents rather than detractors of IQ tests tend to favor it. The training and inclinations of a medical practitioner thus become central to its use or abandonment, reminding us that no cognitive test can be truly objective given that a test measures what a medical practitioner wants to measure, rather than provides an understanding of ASD independent from human prejudices. This defect is central to the human experience because one person's reality differs from all others even when variations are small. The test tends to be used on people with ASD with solid language and mathematical skills. Moreover it appears to be used regularly on adults. The frequency of use cannot be quantified, but a December 2001 article in *Wired*, a monthly magazine that examines technology's effects on American society, drew attention to it and may have increased its popularity.

Other tests purport to focus on so called "real life" skills. In this case the measurer may turn to the adaptive behavior profile. This approach makes sense given that daily existence requires everyone, with ASD or otherwise, to solve concrete problems. Expectations are that people with ASD will score lower on this test than will neurotypical people. Partisans assert that the test reliably documents that an ASD person's ability to cope with the ordinariness of daily life almost always trails his or her intellectual abilities. Such findings are useful to the social worker who wants to help a person with ASD integrate into society. A U.S. National Library of Medicine publication states that, but does explain why, scientists and medical practitioners seldom use the profile. The article asserts that it may reveal information about high functioning people with ASD.

Returning momentarily to the Wechsler scale, its language assessments are similar to specific communication profiles for children who range from an inability to speak to noteworthy fluency. Medical practitioners tend to use them to supplement clinical observations. In this context, no test supersedes careful observation. As hinted earlier, no competent social worker, nurse, or physician pretends that any test or series of tests can yield a complete understanding of ASD.

Even within the context of a priori knowledge, a term defined in detail in a later chapter, cognition is difficult to confine to a person's interior thoughts because it is an active process that interacts with the environment such that outside stimuli affect mental processes. For example, a student's generous self assessment depends at least partly on how others perceive him. In other words and in imitation of the first example, a pianist is gifted not just because of her pyrotechnical abilities but because critics praise her without reservation. With these instances understood, sensory and motor profiles attempt to quantify how someone understands and responds, through the senses, to the outside world. These tests, for example vision and hearing screenings, necessitate measurements of sensory acuity.

ASD FROM OTHER PERSPECTIVES

Important as is the patient, a medical practitioner may consult others to supplement what she has learned through inquiry and observation. Particularly valuable are the parents or, in their absence, the most intimate caregivers. In some cases grandparents or other close kin fulfill this role, but in other cases care falls to adoptive parents or others who are not related to the patient. Biological relatedness is not critical here because what matters most is that the caregiver has a sustained and intimate relationship with the patient. In this regard the caregiver functions as a primary source of information about the patient. Historians have long emphasized that the best information about a person, movement, or event comes from those who have firsthand knowledge about it, with any firsthand account necessarily a primary source. Medical practitioners apply this principle in interviewing caregivers. Such an interview need not be a formal or rigid exchange of information. In many cases a doctor or surrogate asks caregivers the questions that come to mind, modifying subsequent queries in light of new information, making an interview a dynamic and fluid event requiring skill and agility from the doctor. He or she gathers necessary information about the patient without relentlessly probing the caregiver.

In other cases a medical practitioner gathers information through a set of standard questions that supplement knowledge gained informally. Such a tool is the childhood autism rating scale. The questions appeal to doctors who want to gather information through a variety of approaches. For example, parents may complete the questions with little or no guidance from a social worker, nurse, or physician. In other cases, the interviewer, being attuned to the fact that caregivers may dislike a pencil and paper questionnaire because it can evoke unpleasant memories of the high stakes standardized tests they took in school, may ask the questions in an effort to make them as natural as possible. No hard data exist to quantify how often the scale is used, but the Children's Hospital of Philadelphia states that a new version, the childhood autism rating scale-2, has superseded the original.

Other standardized questionnaires include the autism diagnostic interview and the autism diagnostic observation schedule. These instruments have their place when used judiciously, but experts know not to rely too much on them because of their tendency to permit only a limited range of answers. (Such limits are unavoidable because no questionnaire can truly be exhaustive in light of the reality that no one can hope to finish any test that aims to be comprehensive.) Yet these limits are vexing because the questionnaires can never hope to capture the vastness of ASD's signs and symptoms. A list of standard questions risks treating signs and symptoms uniformly, contradicting the reality that ASD varies from person to person. In sum, a medical practitioner pursues the flexibility inherent in any human interaction to counteract the robotic nature of standardized questionnaires.

Emphasis on careful questioning and observation should not disguise the hope that medicine may someday develop a test to identify a biological marker or markers for ASD. It is natural to hope for progress on this front, but medicine cannot guarantee the rapid development of such a test. Remembering the importance of genes in determining ASD's onset and severity, scientists and doctors hope to develop a test to identify faulty genes (genes with one or more mutations). Yet medicine must progress substantially to achieve this goal because, as was mentioned in chapter 3, a large number of genes determine ASD's magnitude. Without their identification no test is in the offing. Even identification does not equal success because scientists and physicians do not fully understand how every gene functions and especially how clusters of genes modify a gene or other genes (Shannon 2011).

BIOLOGICAL ASSESSMENTS OF ASD

A larger point may be in order. An emphasis on genes is necessarily a focus on the genotype. Recall from chapter 3 that the genotype is the total number of genes that one inherits and that only a fraction of these genes operates in a person. Later chapters will enlarge this definition, but such matters do not concern this discussion. Returning to gene function, only active genes matter because only they determine a person's traits. To borrow an analogy from baseball, only the players on the field can win or lose a game. Everyone in the dugout is just a spectator. True, the manager makes decisions, many of them consequential, but he cannot determine the outcome; the burden falls solely on the players who execute his instructions. Retreading the path from genes to traits, the sum of all physical attributes is the phenotype; ASD's signs and symptoms can be observed only because they are the phenotype's physical expressions. In other words, as important as genes are, progress against ASD likely depends more on study of the phenotype than on a singular focus on the genotype, even as no researcher would discount the study of genes as basic to almost every inquiry into an organism's biology. Scientists and physicians continue to pursue such knowledge even when it does not immediately solve a problem. The history of science is replete with examples of knowledge that was not immediately practical but that became useful upon discovery of additional information. (The sagas of antibiotics and microwave ovens merely scratch the surface of this reality.)

A focus on biology, even when it alone cannot diminish ASD's signs and symptoms, nevertheless yields vital information. In this regard, scientists and physicians use neurological assessments to gauge ASD's magnitude. Some tests are obvious and easy to administer. For example, the fact that ASD's cognitive impairments are more prevalent among people with small heads than among people with heads of average size leads medical practitioners to measure the skull's circumference as a way of correlating size with ASD's severity. Recall from chapter 3 that a skull smaller than average houses a brain smaller than average and that a small brain may have limited cognitive abilities. In other words, a small brain, being underdeveloped, tends to display underdeveloped cognition.

These perils are plain, but a brain larger than average may also cause some ASD signs and symptoms. It is thought that an extra-large brain, having too many neurons and synapses, is less efficient than a brain of average size. That is, the greater the number of neurons, the greater appears to be the probability that they may misfire or fire inefficiently. Such problems appear to be central to understanding at least some ASD instances. The dangers of inordinate enlargement are plain in adolescence, when an average brain hastens the process of pruning, during which it reduces the number of synapses while retaining the number of neurons. This consolidation appears to streamline the brain's efficiency. But adolescents whose brain delays and slows pruning lose consolidation's efficiencies. Just as a brain smaller than average causes a condition known as microcephaly, a brain larger than average causes a condition known as macrocephaly. Deviations from the norm in either direction cause at least some ASD problems.

Macrocephaly seems to be at the root of conditions that overlap with ASD, including Sotos syndrome, which appears to arise from an enlarged face and sometimes other parts of the body (often known as gigantism), peculiar body features especially in the face, clumsiness, and cognitive impairments. Comments throughout this book emphasize that cognitive deficits plague severe ASD cases. Chapter 3 noted that some people with ASD have fragile X syndrome, which correlates with macrocephaly. Here again is the specter of cognitive impairment. Macrocephaly may be apparent by age two, though the worst problems usually beset adolescence because of delayed and slow pruning. Because the focus in macrocephaly is on the number of neurons and in adolescence on the number of synapses, the physician may use a technology known as magnetic resonance imaging (MRI) to derive an image of the brain. MRI is another example of advances in pure science that were not immediately useful but that led to its later invention.

For reference, pure science seeks knowledge for its own sake whereas applied science seeks only knowledge that immediately impacts the world. These impacts are generally thought to benefit everyone (at least potentially), as when agronomists bred new varieties of high protein wheat, rice, or corn. But such impacts rarely receive ubiquitous praise because some people fear agricultural improvements, like new types of disease or herbicide resistant soybeans, corn, potatoes, canola, and other crops that come from biotechnology.

Also apparent by age two is hypotonia or subnormal muscle tone, which can weaken toddlers in many ways including lessening balance and coordination. Although the brain region responsible for this condition has not been pinpointed, scientists and doctors believe that hypotonia results from a brain abnormality or abnormalities. It may improve after age two. Perhaps maturation heightens physical activity, thereby improving muscle tone. Attention on hypotonia leads doctors to gauge muscle tone in gathering evidence for an ASD diagnosis. Like brain circumference measurements, evaluations of muscle tone require no sophisticated and expensive technology. Note that hypotonia is not ubiquitous because only about 6 percent of children with ASD have it.

Another piece in ASD's puzzle and its diagnosis is dyspraxia. Recall from chapter 1 dyspraxia's unusual clumsiness in some people with ASD. Like hypotonia, it tends to persist throughout childhood but may decline in adulthood and so demands early evaluation. Again, as in previous examples, diagnosis follows from inspection rather than from special technologies. Diagnosis may be as simple as asking a possible child with ASD to pick up and hold a pen. Failure may unmask dyspraxia and heighten the probability of ASD. This clumsiness may also appear in speech so that the physician need only talk with the patient to strengthen or weaken suspicions of dyspraxia and ASD. As with other conditions, dyspraxia may result from the brain's poorly coordinated neural activity.

Separate from dyspraxia are conditions collectively labeled movement disorders. These problems' breadth prevents recitation of every sign and symptom, but tics, speech abnormalities, and general lapses in coordination may point to these disorders. Because these abnormalities, like some other problems, overlap with ASD, they may contribute to an ASD diagnosis. Again, this diagnosis may be reached through visual and auditory inspections that require no sophisticated technologies. The physician may again talk with the patient to move toward an ASD diagnosis. Alternatively he or she may watch for tics to strengthen suspicions of Tourette's syndrome, another ASD comorbidity.

Recall from earlier chapters that epilepsy may be another comorbidity. The overlap between ASD and epilepsy is only partial because a majority of people with ASD do not have epilepsy. The number cannot be pinpointed, but various studies estimate that between 5 and 40 percent of people with ASD have epilepsy. A good counterexample is the nineteenth century Russian novelist Fyodor Dostoyevsky. Biographers have established his epilepsy though none has speculated that he had ASD. Note the great difficulty in diagnosing ASD posthumously because clinical observations of behavior and other features are no longer possible.

Other paths toward an ASD diagnosis may be traveled; all cannot be trod here, though the somatosensory "road" may be worth a long look. This system, which includes the brain and other parts of the CNS, interprets tactile (touch) sensations. It is fascinating and perhaps bizarre to consider that ASD may reduce or eliminate these sensations. For example, a neurotypical child learns not to touch a hot object because pain results. But pain's absence may endanger a child with ASD who, unaware that a hot object is truly hot, may severely burn him or herself by touching or holding it. This lack of tactile sensation may cause or worsen self injurious behaviors (SIB) in some people with ASD. No responsible physician would ask a patient to touch a hot object as a diagnostic test but would instead ask a caregiver to recollect instances of pain insensitivity or subnormal sensitivity. Also important will be a caregiver's documentation of the patient's SIB, evidence that may pave the road toward an ASD diagnosis.

TREATMENT AND MANAGEMENT

As mentioned earlier, ASD has no cure now so that healthcare professionals must focus on treating its signs and symptoms. In other words, absent a cure, ASD might be managed through a combination of therapeutic drugs, diet and lifestyle changes, and behavioral therapy, all being types of treatment. These options or treatments have outcomes that vary from one patient to another, and an ASD individual's treatment will be unique and may take years of trial and error to develop. Note that treatment and management are not synonymous and that both pivot about the presence or absence of a cure, as implied earlier. When a cure is possible, treatment can achieve it. For example, the antibiotic streptomycin can cure the bacterial infection tuberculosis. But when cure is impossible, treatment can only alleviate or manage signs and symptoms, today's reality for ASD and other conditions including some cancers. In fact, incurability is fundamental to the human condition because of death's inevitability.

A glance at possible treatments or therapies reveals many options. The pharmaceutical industry offers several drugs, many of which were originally developed to treat other conditions. Dietary modifications are numerous, though one wonders about these variants' effectiveness, especially when self promotion is evident and repetitious. Several talk therapies and manipulations of the learning environment have cycled in and out of vogue in the quest to manage ASD. This section cannot hope to exhaust these options, but prominent therapies merit attention.

Drug Therapies

This chapter and earlier ones note that the brain and the rest of the CNS play a large role in ASD, making pharmaceutical options the starting point for treatment because they target the brain and CNS at large. These options depend at least partly on knowledge about serotonin, a chemical the body produces for a range of activities. The brain and gastrointestinal tract produce most of it, which is synthesized from the amino acid tryptophan and a closely related chemical. Scientists know the product as 5-hydroxyltryptamine whereas the lay reader is more familiar with the name serotonin. Variously classified as hormone or neurotransmitter, serotonin regulates the transmission of electrochemical signals between neurons, sets a person's mood, regulates the movement and elimination of wastes, causes nausea when a person eats or drinks a toxin, causes osteoporosis when in excess, regulates the libido, and helps blood clots form.

Its presence in the brain and regulation of mood focus attention on its role in lessening depression. Inadequate serotonin in the brain correlates with depression, though it is unclear whether reductions in serotonin cause depression or depression causes the body to reduce production of serotonin. Popular writers may term this conundrum an instance of the chicken and egg dilemma. Whatever serotonin's role in depression, this correlation has led scientists and physicians to scrutinize it. This observation has led researchers to seek ways to increase serotonin levels in depressed people, leading to the discovery and use of what are known as selective serotonin reuptake inhibitors (SSRI). These carbon based molecules, synthesized in the laboratory, do not stop the brain from producing serotonin but instead impair the brain's ability to reabsorb (reuptake) it. Because the brain absorbs less of the serotonin it produces, more is available to help transmit electrochemical signals between neurons, an apparent benefit to depressed people generally. As many as one third of people with ASD may have too much serotonin in the brain. Because excess brain serotonin seems to benefit depressed people, depressed people with ASD in this category should not need additional help; yet the situation is fluid because some seem to benefit from SSRI whereas others do not. As early as 2010 an Australian scientist at the University of New South Wales and Sydney Children's Hospital in Randwick published her recommendations against SSRI use in a child or adult with ASD given the lack of convincing evidence in their favor. The U.S. National Library of Medicine classifies SSRI as antidepressants, noting their use in roughly 32 percent of children and adults with ASD who also have anxiety. These studies taken together imply that insufficient evidence exists to know how often SSRI are prescribed to treat people with ASD because of depression rather than another comorbidity like anxiety.

These ambiguities are not always in play when profits are apparent. That is, if the development of one inhibitor profits a pharmaceutical firm, others will follow. Consequently the physician may choose among several inhibitors given the common sense approach that if one does little to treat an ASD sign or symptom, another might be tried in hopes of better results, and because side effects may be less severe than with other types of antidepressants. All inhibitors cannot receive space in this chapter, but fluvoxamine deserves mention because it appears to control repetitious behaviors and speech and to reduce aggression, particularly in adults. Recall that repetition and aggression plague some children and adults with ASD.

A similar agent, fluoxetine, appears to minimize repetition and irritability. When it works well, people with ASD are less prone to injure themselves and act aggressively. Repeated use, however, may cause unpleasant side effects like restlessness, hyperactivity, agitation, loss of appetite, or insomnia. Patients seem to benefit from fluoxetine only during treatment. Upon cessation, harmful behaviors return. This situation applies to other drugs and the maladies they treat. For example, discontinuation of blood pressure medicines may elevate blood pressure in patients who have not eliminated harmful habits like eating too much saturated fat.

Another option may be the inhibitor sertraline, though clinical trials have proceeded slowly. It may be too early for optimism, but the small number of studies seems to indicate sertraline's value in reducing aggression and repetition. Better established may be paroxetine, which may reduce SIB, aggression, irritability, tantrums, and lapses in concentration. Its use in cognitively impaired people with ASD appears to be increasing. The inhibitor citalopram may lessen aggression, anxiety, and unhelpful actions and thoughts. Escitalopram may decrease irritability, but otherwise its utility is questionable, especially because a side effect is irritability, in which case the inhibitor worsens the condition it was meant to treat. Again, history is replete with such instances. For example, some people gain rather than lose weight while taking diet pills. Hyperactivity may be another side effect of diet pills.

Another class of drugs includes anticonvulsants and mood stabilizers. These agents are potent, requiring close monitoring. Anticonvulsants have shown promise in treating epilepsy, and the overlap between it and ASD has extended their use to people with ASD. These anticonvulsants may help treat the roughly 30 percent of people with ASD with periodic seizures. Children below age 5 appear to be especially prone to such seizures and are candidates for anticonvulsants.

As with SSRI, research on anticonvulsants has yielded a variety of drugs including valproate, whose versatility extends to treatment of seizures, mania in bipolar people, and migraines. It appears to stabilize moods in people with ASD, though researchers are unsure how to explain any of its benefits, a circumstance common to many other medicines. One line of thought suggests that valproate may lessen the body's production of gamma aminobutyric acid (GABA). Recall from the previous chapter that GABA is a chemical that helps regulate wakefulness and sleepiness. In this context, valproate may reduce the amount of GABA in the body enough to dull sensations of wakefulness and sleepiness in a way that evens out moods. The mechanism of this action is not understood. Another hypothesis holds that valproate may lessen the amount of N-methyl-D-aspartic acid (NMDA), a chemical in nerves that has various critical functions. For reasons that are not understood, a small reduction in NMDA appears to lessen the severity of neurological conditions, among them ASD. Other studies cite valproate's possible effects on neurotransmitters in the belief that the drug improves transmission of electrochemical signals from neuron to neuron. Alternatively, valproate may improve the function of genes that in a suboptimal state increase ASD's severity. All these possibilities need additional research for the medical community to understand how it works.

Like valproate, lamotrigine (brand name lamictal) has various uses including treatment of epilepsy and bipolarity. Epileptic people with ASD benefit from it, according to the National Center for Biotechnology Research in Bethesda, Maryland, and those with ASD and bipolar disorder may take lamotrigine to even out moods, thereby minimizing unpleasant outbursts. Lamotrigine appears to benefit children with ASD, who may be better able to concentrate, socialize, and remain alert. Those with Rett syndrome, a chromosomal condition mentioned in chapter 3, may benefit the most from lamotrigine. As with several other drugs, lamotrigine's mechanisms of action mystify scientists and physicians and demand more research. Another option is levetiracetam, a drug with a different chemistry than valproate or lamotrigine. It appears to help people with ASD who have epilepsy in ways that are not understood. Levetiracetam may decrease the activity of two chemicals in the cerebellum, thereby reducing excitability, agitation, and aggression in people with ASD who are prone to outbursts.

Topiramate, like a handful of other drugs, lessens the severity of seizures in ASD people with epilepsy. It appears to help comorbid children and adults and may be better than antipsychotics like risperidone in averting weight gain, particularly in children. Some children and adults, with or without ASD, lose rather than gain weight, though the loss is usually small enough not to worry parents or physicians. Nonetheless, as much as one fifth of children and adults with ASD lose enough weight to cause the doctor to discontinue topiramate. Even under the best circumstances, it may heighten agitation, irritability, and hyperactivity. In this context, part of medicine's art is the ability to balance potential rewards against risks to achieve the best outcome.

Carbamazepine may treat seizures and stabilize moods in people with ASD. Like many other drugs, carbamazepine baffles scientists and doctors who want to know why it works. Hypotheses abound as some researchers posit that carbamazepine regulates production of GABA and serotonin, both having been mentioned earlier. Others think that carbamazepine improves how the hippocampus and cortex function in people with ASD. Possibly valuable in managing ASD, carbamazepine has had few clinical trials because it causes seizures in some patients. Chemically similar to carbamazepine, oxcarbamazepine also treats seizures and stabilizes moods in people with ASD. As its name suggests, oxcarbamazepine has one more oxygen atom than carbamazepine and has the same actions and risks. As with carbamazepine, researchers hesitate to test oxcarbamazepine in clinical trials of people with ASD.

Any discussion of mood stabilizers must mention lithium, a soft metal on the periodic table and one so reactive that it does not exist unbounded in nature. In a medical context, lithium often binds with carbonate ions to form the drug lithium carbonate. In this form, lithium has been a much prescribed and studied mood stabilizer. It benefits some patients with various ailments. Even with widespread use, lithium has received few clinical trials in people with ASD. An August 2014 report available online at the

National Center of Biotechnology Information notes that lithium trials are promising enough to justify further research. Because lithium helps stabilize moods it may treat aggression, irritability, and agitation in people with ASD. Case studies extend these benefits to both children and adults with ASD.

Other types of drugs are available. One important class is the antipsychotic. Recall that a psychosis causes a person to perceive the outside world in ways that a nonpsychotic person does not such that a psychotic person inhabits a distorted reality. Medicines known as antipsychotics, initially developed to treat psychotic people, have gained attention during the last 50 years as agents to lessen ASD signs and symptoms, particularly in children. As with other classes of drugs, several antipsychotics are on the market.

One antipsychotic, clozapine, may treat aggression in people with ASD, particularly children. This hope hangs by slender threads, being derived from a small study. In another case, clozapine improved sociability and lessened repetitive behaviors in one man. These successes, limited to just these case studies, occurred without side effects, a rare circumstance for any drug. The elimination of side effects is implausible given clozapine's potential to make patients with ASD sleepy or put them at risk for seizures. More research is needed to clarify these issues.

Earlier was mentioned risperidone, which the U.S. Food and Drug Administration (FDA) has approved to treat ASD signs and symptoms, including irritability, in children with ASD between ages five and sixteen. Researchers have studied its effects in adults with ASD, noting some success against irritability, repetitive behaviors, aggression, anxiety, and depression. Adults with ASD deficient in sociability and language appear not to benefit from risperidone. Drowsiness is a side effect; other potential problems are not yet apparent.

Another option is the antipsychotic olanzapine, which treats aggression and anxiety in ways similar to those of certain other drugs. It appears to improve sociability, though weight gain is a risk, particularly because the increase may be large. In trials, sedation emerged as the principal side effect. Side effects, particularly weight gain, have lessened olanzapine's appeal in managing ASD. Olanzapine is not unique because many antipsychotics as well as many antidepressants cause patients to gain weight.

The antipsychotic quetiapine yields inconsistent results. Some clinical trials have detected improvements in some ASD signs and symptoms, though subjects are no more social while taking it. In other cases, seizures have marred the potential for improvements. Also worrisome are side effects that include aggression, agitation, increased weight, and sleepiness, prompting researchers to discontinue trials.

Ziprasidone, a widely prescribed antipsychotic, appears to work much like the previously mentioned SSRI and may lessen aggression, agitation, and irritability. Sleepiness is a side effect, but ziprasidone is unusual among antipsychotics in promoting weight loss, though close monitoring is necessary to avoid losses that are too large. Clinical trials confirm that about 80 percent of patients with ASD lose weight, an effect notable upon switching from an antipsychotic that promotes weight gain to ziprasidone. Reductions in blood cholesterol sometimes accompany weight loss.

The antipsychotic aripiprazole holds promise in ameliorating aggression, impulsiveness, irritability, hyperactivity, and SIB, results noteworthy in children and adolescents. Studies, few in number, suggest that of people with ASD who take aripiprazole, approximately 40 percent can expect to lose weight, 40 percent can expect to maintain weight, and the remaining 20 percent can expect to gain weight. Sleepiness is a side effect, but others appear to be benign. Aripiprazole does not appear to change blood pressure or heart rate.

Dietary Therapies

Drug therapies are not the only option. Some health enthusiasts want people with ASD to minimize or eliminate gluten from the diet. Gluten is a complex of proteins common in wheat (including durum), rye, barley, and triticale. All are grasses classified more narrowly as grains, though others, notably oats and rice, lack gluten. Gluten gives the flour of wheat, rye, barley, and triticale the stickiness necessary for making bread.

Some people poorly tolerate gluten, and those with celiac disease cannot eat foods containing it without becoming ill. These facts lead some nutritionists, dieticians, and kindred professionals to advise all consumers to minimize or eliminate it from the diet. If this rationale makes sense for all people, then those with ASD should likewise adopt this practice. As logical as this advice may appear to be, studies have detected no benefits from minimizing or reducing gluten in hopes of lessening ASD's signs and symptoms. The foregoing does not eliminate the possibility that people with ASD might benefit in other ways by eschewing gluten.

Probiotics, microbes that may be introduced into the intestines to improve their function, are also the subject of study and media attention. Such treatments may hold promise against some maladies, but studies about probiotics' uses in people with ASD appear as magazine anecdotes rather than peer reviewed journal articles and so are not on par with clinical data.

Vitamin and mineral supplements have been popular for roughly a century and may be tried in people with ASD. Attention focuses on vitamin C, whose popularity in fighting colds may be found in folklore that predates scientific interest. Perhaps even more attention focuses on the eight B vitamins, especially vitamin B12 (cobalamin) and vitamin B9 (folic acid or folate). The B vitamins help the body convert food into energy. Vitamin B12 is essential in helping the body manufacture red blood cells and in maintaining nerves, functions aided by vitamin B9. Moreover, folic acid helps cells replicate by increasing the manufacture of DNA and RNA, macromolecules defined in previous chapters. Because fetuses, children, adolescents, and pregnant woman all grow rapidly, their cells replicate often and so demand much folic acid. In addition to working with vitamin B12, folic acid also cooperates with vitamin B6 (pyridoxine) to control how much amino acid homocysteine is in blood. This regulation is essential because in high amounts, homocysteine correlates with heart disease. Vitamin supplements may benefit people with ASD with metabolic disorders, but too few studies exist to permit generalizations about how particular vitamins benefit people with ASD. Multivitamins usually contain several minerals in addition to vitamins. These minerals are really metals like iron, calcium, copper, and zinc or nonmetals like phosphorus, which helps form the essential nucleic acids DNA and RNA and is in adenosine triphosphate (ATP), the primary energy source for all life. In other words, consumption of minerals in the right doses benefits all people, including people with ASD.

Another therapy focuses on the inclusion of polyunsaturated fats (like the omega-3 fatty acids in fish) in the diets of neurotypical and people with ASD. Some scientists and physicians hypothesize that people with ASD tend to be deficient in these beneficial fats, but clinical studies fail to confirm the benefits of adding them to the diet. Even were such studies optimistic about polyunsaturated fats, research on children with ASD has produced too few results to permit generalizations. The foregoing should not obscure the fact that polyunsaturated fats appear to benefit people regardless of their medical histories.

Behavioral Therapies

Apart from drugs and diet, other therapies attempt to decrease harmful behaviors in people with ASD. Attention focuses on what are generally known as behavioral therapies, the most studied being applied behavioral analysis therapy (ABA). Practitioners use ABA mostly on children with ASD. Covered more fully in chapter 9, ABA operates on several assumptions, the touchstone being the belief that any attempt to modify behavior should focus solely on practical outcomes. There is little value in theoretical musings. In this sense, all behavioral modifications should be observable, subject to measurement, and permanent.

ABA—originating partly in American behaviorist B. F. Skinner's psychological research, gaining traction in the 1950s, carrying its momentum into the 1980s, and remaining important today—centers on improving quality of life for children with ASD through interventions designed for their utility. ABA may improve sociability even if gains are not breathtaking. The problem lies partly with unscrupulous and undertrained therapists who exaggerate what ABA can hope to achieve per unit time. Such boastfulness dashes parents' hopes for dramatic improvements in their children and adolescents with ASD.

Any discussion of treatment and management must include education, so pervasive an instrument is it in social engineering. Education through grade 12 has been compulsory in the United States for roughly one hundred years. Even though high school graduation is not ubiquitous, enough Americans have experienced public or private schooling to know it intimately. Because Americans tend to believe that anyone can benefit from education, it is unsurprising that compassionate people envision schooling as a way to improve quality of life for children and adolescents with ASD. Extended into adulthood, schooling takes the form of postsecondary education, though many people believe that adults with ASD are suitable for training only in manual occupations like plumbing or carpentry. Theorists have constructed what are known as educational models for ASD individuals. When applied to childhood, the emphasis is on early schooling as the best hope for lasting improvements. This early outreach attempts to capture the attention of children with ASD who otherwise have trouble focusing on a topic for any duration. Once a child is attentive, teachers break a task or concept into small concrete units in the expectation that he or she can master each through hands-on practice at a comfortable pace. The emphasis on mastery seeks proficiency rather than age as the basis for promotion from grade to grade.

CONCLUSION

Diagnosis identifies ASD and initiates treatment in hopes of managing it given that management is the only hope for improving quality of life in someone with an incurable condition. ASD's treatment and management take many forms depending on attributes, inclinations, and competencies of doctor and patient. Therapies include drugs, dietary modifications, behavioral interventions, and education. With ASD's cure probably still distant, medical practitioners continue to pursue objectives like articulating ASD's probable course and complications in hopes of delivering the best care with the least risks to ASD children, adolescents, and adults. The probable outcome, known as the prognosis, joins potential complications as the next chapter's focus.

REFERENCES

Shannon, Joyce Brennfleck. 2011. *Autism and Pervasive Developmental Disorders Sourcebook.* 2nd ed. Detroit: Omnigraphics.

6

Long-Term Prognosis and Potential Complications

A prognosis is an attempt to predict the future course of a disease, condition, malady, affliction, ailment, or disorder. No prediction can guarantee an outcome; for example, no prognosis of recovery from a heart attack can guarantee that the patient will not die upon exiting the hospital. This may be extended to the notion of potential complications. A potential complication is some unfortunate circumstance that can occur even when thought improbable. The patient who left the hospital with a clean bill of health might have had such a complication if an undetected blood clot left a vein to lodge in his heart, stopping it and thereby killing him.

Prognosis is necessary for all maladies, especially those like autism spectrum disorder (ASD) that are incurable because a curable affliction's outcome is easier to predict than the course of an incurable problem. To return to an example in the previous chapter, because the antibiotic streptomycin can cure the bacterial infection tuberculosis, cure should be certain given proper administration of the antibiotic and the patient's adherence to all instructions including ingestion of all streptomycin tablets as directed. But conditions like ASD occupy a different universe given that no amount of antibiotics can cure ASD because it is not a bacterial infection. With ASD and kindred problems, a medical practitioner must weigh various factors in arriving at a prognosis. Key to this assessment is a judgment of potential complications. In ASD cases, a physician, nurse, or other expert tries to specify the factors that might harm a child not only early in life but as he or she matures into an adult. An evaluation of potential complications helps a doctor tailor therapies to each ASD patient's needs. Such individualized treatment is important because ASD, as is evident from previous chapters, has many signs and symptoms that vary in onset and severity. In combating this breadth, a medical expert arrives at a set of goals that are pursued in conjunction with an ASD patient in hopes of achieving the best outcome.

PROGNOSIS

Medical Concerns

This book and other literature note that a medical practitioner must labor to lessen ASD's signs and symptoms through various treatments. These treatments manage ASD because they cannot cure it. This approach is common to the many lifelong conditions that beset humans. Consider systemic lupus erythematosus (usually labeled lupus for convenience) or severe depression that may or may not lead to psychotic episodes as examples of lifetime conditions that may be treated but not cured. In the worst cases, treatments fail to manage the patient, who dies after suffering great distress over long intervals. As with these and other examples, the best path toward improvement is early treatment given that some people with ASD are diagnosed at birth. Sometimes telltale ASD signs and symptoms—like low birth weight, microcephaly, or macrocephaly (discussed in chapters 4 and 5)—are present early to confirm this diagnosis. On other occasions, a newborn appears fine only to develop problems like delayed acquisition of language during the first few years of life. Macrocephaly is another example because it may not be apparent at birth. Whatever the signs or symptoms, a physician begins treatment at the earliest opportunity. Treatments fall into one of three categories: cognitive, social, or behavioral. All fall within medicine's purview, though treatments vary within and outside these categories. Previous chapters have surveyed treatment options, including efforts to teach language as early as possible to children with ASD whether neurotypical or cognitively impaired, to direct attention to the external world in socially deficient children and adults through therapies that may involve attempts at socialization in school. Some therapies may try to minimize tantrums and other outbursts through negative feedback including removal of the distraught child from venues that might otherwise interest him or her and positive feedback like hugs, kisses, and other nurturing acts to reward calmness. Chapter 5 details these treatments.

Improvement of signs and symptoms may follow from medical intervention or even neglect given the possibility that they might moderate on their own. Such thinking is not wishful because children with ASD with daunting signs and symptoms may grow into adults better able to manage them. Management comes as much from physical, intellectual, psychological, emotional, spiritual, and social maturation as from an autistic adult's growing ability to disguise what ails him or her. This process is not deceptive because all people occasionally wear masks to shield themselves from stress. The section on employment pursues this reasoning to explain at least partly why some adults with ASD, despite disability, succeed at a job, though such success is not assured because they may encounter barriers that prevent them from securing work in the first place.

Adults with ASD may climb the economic ladder at least partly through success at a university. Livestock expert, author, and lecturer Temple Grandin, mentioned in earlier chapters, exemplifies the success of the most ambitious and industrious people with ASD in higher education. Nonetheless, many people with ASD end their schooling upon graduation from high school, underscoring the need for a treatment plan years before commencement. Sixty-five percent of U.S. students with ASD finish their education upon graduating from high school (Shattuck, et al. 2012). Yet only 58 percent of these students have a treatment plan before or by age fourteen despite the fact that the federal government mandates a plan, whose goals must aim to prepare people with ASD for work after high school, perhaps through volunteering, shadowing, summer work, or internships.

Beyond economic considerations, the plan must prepare people with ASD to live as independently as possible. In the best cases, they live on their own in an apartment or home. In the quest for independence, they learn, through training in high school or in another venue, how to shop at stores, interact with retail associates, bankers, and others encountered in the workaday world, and maintain adequate hygiene and grooming. In other words, socialization emerges as a priority in lessening ASD's long term potential complications. Government agencies in addition to public and private schools may help people with ASD achieve these aims.

Psychological Concerns

Part of ASD treatments to minimize signs and symptoms, and thereby evade long term complications as much as possible, includes management of psychological problems that may originate in self perceptions and that tend to be labeled self esteem issues, a category that is not easy to define. Consider self esteem an interior GPS system that orients a person toward self fulfillment, confidence, and even happiness despite the negative events and stimuli that afflict everyone. In other words, self esteem is a roadmap toward the top of Maslow's hierarchy. Briefly, twentieth century American psychologist Abraham Maslow constructed something akin to a ladder of needs, atop which was self actualization. This language may seem scientific and novel, but at its foundation the hierarchy is a path towards happiness. (Such concerns are not new and go back to fourth century BCE Greek philosopher Aristotle and perhaps even earlier. Moreover, the path toward happiness cannot be straightforward given that Aristotle's celebration of happiness as a noble goal contrasts radically with twentieth century German physicist and Nobel laureate Albert Einstein's conclusion that it is worthy only of pigs.)

Putting aside the difficulties defining happiness and elaborating the GPS analogy, a person who lacks this system may spiral downward into gloom, despair, and disenchantment. If this scenario is true, ASD's potential complication of frail self esteem flows from social deficits. Various behavioral therapies, mentioned in chapter 5, include applied behavioral analysis therapy (ABA), an outgrowth of American psychologist B. F. Skinner's work during the 1930s. In line with his ideas, ABA seeks to elevate the study and modification of behavior into a science subject to analysis and quantification. Believing that the behaviors of a person with ASD, or anyone else, should be predictable and rational (the goals of predictability and rationality being as old as Aristotle's ideas and those of his mentor Plato), ABA acts to reinforce positive behaviors and discourage negative ones. Many therapists in this camp claim to rely on positive reinforcement (known as the carrot) to strengthen beneficial behaviors whereas they style themselves less apt to use negative reinforcement (known as the stick) to discourage maladapted behaviors. Chapter 9 examines these claims in light of strong and numerous criticisms against them. ABA therapists began to seek clients among the parents of children with ASD during the 1960s, touting a variety of approaches including one to one or group counseling, formal classroom instruction, or informal play therapy. The accent is on acquiring practical skills and behaviors like listening, speaking, and reading, emulating role models, and learning to decode others' intentions through studying nonverbal cues. None of these attributes is easy for people with ASD to achieve.

In addition to self esteem is the issue of self absorption (narcissism), a person's preoccupation with himself or herself to the exclusion of others and the tendency to be excessively introspective and introverted. People with ASD may languish in "complete social isolation" (Ewing 2015). Such an individual tends to live in his or her head, if such language is permissible. People with ASD are not alone in being preoccupied with their internal thoughts, but they may be particularly susceptible to this kind of fleeting interaction with the world. Such people are more preoccupied with ideas than objects. Accordingly they may not be adept at learning mechanical skills like the use of a hammer or screwdriver. A May 2009 report by the U.S. National Library of Medicine noted that even high functioning people with ASD seldom display mechanical abilities.

This factor aside, introspection is not always negative. Consider the introspection necessary to achieve the stream of consciousness techniques of noteworthy twentieth century novelists including Irishman James Joyce and American Nobel laureate William Faulkner. But in excess, introspection, introversion, self absorption, and other such tendencies complicate ASD. Inordinate introversion may be difficult to restrain even after treatments requiring years or even a lifetime. As with self-esteem issues, the self-absorbed person with ASD may respond to ABA or another behavioral therapy given sufficient time, commitment, energy, and effort from both therapist and patient (Autism Speaks, n.d.). The study reinforces the sentiment that long term treatments are necessary to combat ASD's potential complications, several having been mentioned earlier. Quick fixes and fad treatments that prey upon patients and caregivers desperate for an illusory cure never work. Dietary treatments like large doses of vitamins C and the B complex as well as the ingestion of copious amounts of omega 3 fatty acids fall into these categories. These nutrients are necessary for health, but this book and kindred studies find no evidence supporting the claim that dietary modifications benefit people with ASD beyond the scope of nutrition.

Social Concerns

Earlier chapters have established that ASD's signs and symptoms include social difficulties. People with ASD, from childhood to adulthood, tend to struggle to forge and sustain relationships, a reality covered in chapter 7. Interactions with peers, family members, coworkers, and authorities pose difficulties for many people with ASD. Socialization problems affect not only people with ASD but caregivers as well.

Caregivers accumulate stress from the demands of raising and interacting with a person with ASD (Benson 2006). Yet both people with ASD and caregivers often lack the social support that might ease their burdens. Mothers more than fathers seem to need social support in raising a child with ASD. In addition, the dearth of social support affects children especially in adolescence. Adolescent boys with ASD need roughly four times more social support than girls with ASD. Teen boys with ASD who receive too little support find themselves lonely (Lasgaard et al. 2010). The loneliest boys lack support from schoolmates, parents, acquaintances, and friends.

Forging and maintaining friendships, crucial for anyone, challenges these boys. Loneliness may impair cognition because the brain needs social stimulation to function well. Loneliness among people with ASD correlates with depression, anxiety, and suicidal tendencies.

This line of thought underscores the dangers of inadequate support from parents. Like all people, those with ASD look to parents for stability, warmth, and nurturing. Many people, including people with ASD, never outgrow this need, and even adults with ASD want tenderness from their parents. Accordingly, absent or inadequate support from parents may harm people with ASD throughout life, even when the parents are no longer alive. Such people with ASD feel guilty, developing the mindset that they are unworthy of parents' love and support (Bishop et al. 2007). Here again, these thoughts may lead to depression, anxiety, and suicidal issues. Where parents are unable to care for children with ASD, the burden sometimes falls on grandparents (Anderson 2010). In these instances, children with ASD seek love and support from their grandparents. Note, however, that the foregoing does not affirm the refrigerator mom thesis discussed in earlier chapters. For reference, this now discredited thesis holds that mothers and surrogates who are cold and distant cause their children to develop ASD.

These problems amplify the isolation that sometimes plagues children with ASD (Lasgaard 2010). Isolation may take many forms in detachment from parents, peers, schoolmates, and others. To combat isolation, many medical practitioners advocate full inclusion of children and adolescents with ASD in school and in the least restrictive environment. The same goal applies to people with ASD who pursue higher education. School is an important vehicle of socialization. Such effects are difficult to duplicate in other ways, magnifying the importance of immersion in the classroom and on the playground at recess. School provides children with ASD, and all children for that matter, an opportunity to interact with peers and adults as they engage with teachers, administrators, aides, and other students.

Part of school socialization involves the pursuit of friendships. Children, adolescents, and adults with ASD experience trouble in this regard at least partly because people with ASD are sometimes unable to distinguish a true friend from someone posing as a friend but who is intent only on using them (Vicker n.d.). In other words, people with ASD can have trouble identifying and avoiding deceptive individuals, the proverbial wolves in sheep's clothing. Central to this problem is the difficulty that some people with ASD have decoding the agenda of others. Uncertainty leads some people with ASD to make bad decisions under duress. Consequently, some people with ASD have difficulty trusting others.

These problems escalate when people brand individuals with ASD odd or weird as though something is inherently wrong with them (Vicker n.d.).

Such negativity lowers self esteem, an issue mentioned earlier. Such branding is tantamount to stigmatization. Unkind thoughts and actions lead children to tease, and in some cases ostracize, their ASD classmates, deepening isolation. Throughout life, people with ASD may be so isolated that they seldom cement meaningful long term relationships.

EMPLOYMENT

Previous chapters have emphasized ASD's early onset. This focus should not deflect attention from the reality that ASD is a lifelong condition that shapes all phases of life including adulthood, a time devoted to earning a living. But in its worst manifestations, ASD prevents more than 60 percent of people with ASD from working (Roux et al. 2015). Without work, they depend on family and the government for financial support and will not be considered in this section, which emphasizes employment. ASD's long term potential complications shape how well or poorly people with ASD perform on the job.

A truism holds that job openings engender fierce competition, and one opening can elicit hundreds of applications. Such competition is not new and seems to affect almost all job seekers. The situation for people with ASD seems particularly daunting, especially when they must compete for work against those lacking a disability or condition. Even in a modern economy, stigma still hinders disabled persons from finding and keeping work.

Under these conditions, some people with ASD need help to maximize their chances of securing work. Alert to the problem, Congress passed the Individuals with Disabilities Education Act (IDEA), originally known as the Education for All Handicapped Children Act, in 1975 and reauthorized it in 1990 and 2004. As the original name suggests, the act focused on children because ASD and like conditions usually appear early in life. The law operates on the premise that schools should give disabled students, including those with ASD, the skills necessary for employment.

Here is the practical approach mentioned earlier in the context of ABA. Given these circumstances, education should help disabled students pivot from school to work and should serve several purposes. First, it should help those with ASD and other disabilities (for simplicity, this section refers to "people with ASD" in lieu of repeating the phrase "people with ASD and others with disabilities") learn about the breadth of jobs. Second, education should help people with ASD gauge their abilities and proclivities. A dose of realism is necessary because some students, and not just people with ASD, will never learn the mathematics necessary to become an engineer. Once schools have helped people with ASD concretize abilities and aspirations, they should provide training necessary to secure relevant work. But the K-12 system may take students only partly toward this goal. In the case of high functioning people with ASD (once known as people with Asperger's syndrome), a university education may be necessary to impart the applicable skills. Having secured training appropriate to abilities and interests, people with ASD must fulfill other requirements including how to get to work and return home after their shift. High functioning people with ASD may have a driver's license and a car. Others rely on public transportation because it is less stressful than the arduous driving in traffic or bad weather. Solving these problems does not guarantee a smooth transition from unemployment to work. Those with internships, summer jobs, or volunteer experience may be able to compete for employment.

Worldwide nonprofit Lime Connect lists numerous job openings and internships to help disabled people secure work, usually their first job, at www.limeconnect.com. These positions are not bottom feeders but rather come from technology companies willing to pay well for technical and mathematical abilities, strengths of some ASD job seekers. Incidentally, the phrase "entry level job" is falling out of favor because almost all jobs now require experience and so cannot lead to work at the lowest levels of skills and performance.

People with ASD who benefit from IDEA may still encounter problems, at least partly because few schools provide additional avenues for employment exploration after graduation. Government agencies like the state bureaus of vocational rehabilitation labor to fill the void by helping people with ASD and other disabled people find work. These agencies provide a variety of services, including aptitude and ability testing, identification of suitable career clusters, assistance applying for employment, and help interviewing for a job, all without charge to the participant. Sometimes these agencies assign a person with ASD his or her own job counselor. Such an approach is labor intensive and costly so is short term. Depending on its timetable, an agency may discharge a person with ASD who has not found work within six months.

Types of Jobs

Throughout employment explorations, a person with ASD might investigate opportunities within three tiers (Holtz, Owings, and Ziegert 2006). Jobs requiring the least skills (first tier) are known as segregated or secured. The term "segregated" refers to the likelihood that employers will assign a new ASD hire to work alongside other people with ASD. In such cases a person with ASD does not compete against neurotypicals to secure a job or to complete tasks once hired. Such jobs do not offer prestige because they seldom require advanced skills or allot high pay and benefits. Accordingly they attract people with ASD with the greatest deficits who nonetheless can work.

The second tier is known as supported. In this category, a worker with ASD receives some level of support to help him or her perform well. This support may include careful supervision from a manager or team leader, a circumstance that sometimes worries these employees afraid of rebuke. The Forward Motion Coaching email newsletters, tailored to high functioning people with ASD and those with similar developmental issues, detail these problems. Support may also come from the aforementioned state bureaus of vocational rehabilitation. Bureau agents who assist disabled clients prepare them to function with the least supervision, benefiting both employee and employer. The best outcomes enable disabled people like people with ASD to excel even without supervision. This second tier integrates people with ASD into the workforce such that they work and interact with neurotypical coworkers.

The third level is known as competitive because people with ASD compete with neurotypicals on an equal footing and from the outset. This level expects immediate integration into the workforce. In this arena an employee with ASD comes to a job with skills that allow him or her to meet an employer's every expectation. These abilities may not include the soft skills on display in delicate interpersonal dealings with coworkers. Rather they may be hard skills such as mathematical and computer competencies that technology companies value. As noted above, Lime Connect posts such jobs and internships online. Such skilled workers command pay, status, and benefits on par with neurotypical coworkers, though such perks fail to ensnare the many nonmaterialistic people with ASD (Holtz, Owings, and Ziegert 2006). Rather than lavish compensation, they seek work that enriches them irrespective of pay.

The Work Environment

These considerations demonstrate that people with ASD, like their neurotypical counterparts, need work that fulfills their expectations in a variety of ways. The worker with ASD needs a job that matches interests, abilities, hours, quest for status or pay where applicable, amount of interpersonal interactions, benefits, and other applicable perks (Holtz, Owings, and Ziegert 2006). Attention must focus on the physical environment given the perils of overstimulation because workers with ASD dislike too much noise and artificial light. For example, a high functioning person with ASD may write satisfactory prose but nevertheless be a poor journalist because of the typical newsroom's commotion and noise. Freelance assignments might be a better option, even when pay is meager, if they can be completed in silence at home. The foregoing does not eliminate journalism as a possible career. Temple Grandin (2017), herself a person with ASD and accomplished writer, describes high functioning people with ASD who excel in journalism because of the discipline and structure they learned as children.

Workers with ASD who use and interpret language literally benefit from a supervisor's clear expectations (Standifer 2009). Return to the example of writers with ASD who benefit, as all writers do, from an ironclad deadline. They tend to break a deadline into its component parts, facilitating the daily completion of the number of words that, when summed over the assignment's duration, meet the deadline. When this regimen is inflexible, a writer with ASD may not retire for the night until meeting and sometimes exceeding the daily goal. To ask for an extension is tantamount to a declaration of failure for a writer with ASD (Woog n.d.; Boucher and Oehler 2013).

Viewing workers with ASD, especially those in the first tier of jobs, as inadequate minimizes their strengths, which include fixation on completing tasks on time. To this benefit may be added their reliability (Wallis 2012). A job that begins at 8 a.m. marks the start of work such that people with ASD will not arrive at 8:02. Delay requires them to seek a supervisor's forgiveness and to arrive at 7:58 the next day. Reliability is especially valuable in occupations considered undesirable. For example, the fast food industry seldom attracts the most reliable workers. Here people with ASD shine because they do not call off work at the last moment or fail to appear at the appointed time. Attending to details, a dishwasher with ASD will clean dishes such that they are suitable for immediate use without rewashing because of stray food particles.

The example of a dishwasher, confined to a backroom and segregated from others, highlights another facet, namely that workers with ASD may feel uncomfortable in positions requiring interaction with the public (Standifer 2009). Returning to journalism, ASD writers may be uncomfortable meeting and interviewing public officials and similar people, reinforcing the notion that journalism may not appeal to them.

Yet this stipulation may not be a drawback. Uncomfortable among groups, a person with ASD may instead excel in relative isolation. For example, workers with ASD may shine as computer programmers at least partly because they are able to sit all day in front of a computer, concentrating their full attention on the task (Holtz, Owings, and Ziegert 2006). Such workers seldom need hands on supervision because they manage time and follow directions with painstaking precision, all the while tracking details. Returning to journalism, ASD writers meet editorial needs by delivering a 1000-word article on or before deadline and very near the word limit.

An article that requires five illustrations will fill the inbox with additional ones, allowing editors to select those most suitable for the magazine.

Expecting an orderly flow of events during the day, workers with ASD may not be adept at multitasking, the modern economy's principle watchword. Temple Grandin confirmed the managerial belief that workers with ASD cannot multitask (Adams 2010). What might appear to be a shortcoming is not truly problematic because people with ASD partition an assignment into a linear sequence of tasks completed in order with what might be described as robotic precision. These workers fit the specifications of employers who dislike holding employees' hands all day while they vacillate between ideas and indecision. As for multitasking, it may be a misnomer because rarely can someone complete two tasks at once, though it may be possible to complete two tasks in rapid succession. (Such frankness does not contradict the workaday world in which anyone who has had to avoid an errant car because of the driver's mindless cell phone chatter knows that the notion of multitasking fails to square with reality.)

With all that a worker with ASD offers, the real challenge is securing work in the first place. The habit of pigeonholing job candidates and employees according to preconceptions gives the human resources department great latitude in determining who is or is not qualified for a job. People with ASD must therefore convince the human resources manager and colleagues that they merit an interview. The first step in this process is tailoring a résumé and cover letter to the job advertisement's specifications. But the posting is itself a barrier because ASD applicants seldom apply unless they meet or exceed every requirement. Such literal thinking is a liability whenever human resources seeks an applicant who satisfies most but not all criteria because of the preconception that someone who meets all requirements will become bored with the job. People with ASD who apply for a job may excel on paper because they fastidiously fit a resume and cover letter to the job's requirements. This skill may get them an interview, where the real challenge becomes apparent. Grandin has emphasized the importance of selling skills not personality. Her success as writer, lecturer, and academic makes difficult any temptation to dismiss this advice as unrealistic, but too strict an adherence to it backfires whenever human resources hires the charismatic candidate over the most qualified one, a reality of the corporate world. Such thinking disqualifies socially inept ASD job seekers.

POTENTIAL COMPLICATIONS

Potential complications are emphasized throughout this chapter and take various forms. Physical problems harm people with ASD in multiple ways. Earlier chapters note the correlation between ASD and epilepsy and other seizure disorders. Chapter 4 notes that sensory problems like deafness and tactile deficits plague people with ASD. Metabolic and endocrine problems, chief among them diabetes, afflict people with ASD. Allergies or asthma are common, and obesity contributes to diabetes and heart disease, both of which, as has been mentioned, trouble adults with ASD and the aged and shorten lives. Cerebral palsy, a cluster of movement disorders arising during childhood, disables some people with ASD. As noted in chapter 1, some people with ASD suffer from constipation.

Other ASD potential complications include mental disorders, but because they arise in the brain, they too are physical even though convention puts them in a separate category. This habit arises from labeling such issues as psychological. The noun "psychology" has roots in another noun, "psyche," which was long synonymous with soul, spirit, or some unspecified metaphysical element. Earlier chapters note the prevalence of cognitive deficits, sometimes termed mental retardation, in ASD's worst cases. Apart from such deficits, people with ASD may suffer from depression, anxiety, unstable moods, and suicidal thoughts and actions, problems resulting from chemical imbalances in the brain. Recalling from past chapters the notion that biology and environment together shape people, these twin elements interact to determine the severity of depression, anxiety, and similar problems.

Among mental disorders exists the problem, apparent in the nineteenth century and noted in chapter 2, of distinguishing between ASD and schizophrenia. Recall that schizophrenia does not cause multiple personalities, a psychosis known as dissociative identity disorder or multiple personality disorder and described in the June 2008 issue of the journal *Current Psychiatry Reports*. Instead, schizophrenia is a brain disorder that causes other kinds of psychoses in the sufferer. Schizophrenics typically have trouble thinking and concentrating and may be withdrawn or unmotivated. As early as the 1940s, clinicians noted overlap between signs and symptoms in ASD (then known as autism) and schizophrenia. Among them, Austrian American physician and autism pioneer Leo Kanner, mentioned in chapter 2, had trouble distinguishing between ASD and schizophrenia. Current research documents that the connection is more than clinical because both are rooted in biology, a theme recurrent in this book and other literature.

As biological phenomena, ASD and schizophrenia both appear to involve the brain's cortex. Recall that the cortex is the cerebrum's outermost layer and endows humans with consciousness. One or more genes that guide the cortex's development are likely faulty in both people with ASD and schizophrenics. Collaboration among the University of Iowa Carver College of Medicine in Iowa City, Johns Hopkins University in Baltimore, Maryland, and Cold Spring Harbor Laboratory in Cold Spring

Harbor, New York, has identified 84 faulty genes that may cause both ASD and schizophrenia. These genes may also play a role in bipolar disorder's onset and severity, linking all three conditions.

CONCLUSION

With no cure in sight, ASD is a lifelong condition whose prognosis forecasts unremitting treatment to lessen signs and symptoms and avert potential complications that mar a person with ASD's life. Medical concerns include epilepsy and other seizure disorders, allergies, asthma, constipation, sensory deficits, obesity, diabetes, heart disease, cerebral palsy, cognitive deficiencies, unstable moods, depression, anxiety, suicidal thoughts and actions, and related issues. Attention focuses on links between ASD and schizophrenia and ranges far to examine the difficulties of finding and keeping a job. Emphasis was placed on the social deficits that beget long term complications like the employment difficulties just noted. These deficits define ASD and complicate attempts to interact with caregivers (whether parents, grandparents, or guardians), peers, schoolmates, and potential friends. Throughout this chapter the school, ranging from pre kindergarten to terminal or professional degree, emerges as an important social setting for children, adolescents, and adults with ASD, providing opportunities for interactions with classmates, teachers, and others in a variety of contexts; yet the school has problems wherever classmates brand people with ASD as odd or weird, reinforcing the tendency to stigmatize and ostracize them. People with ASD have difficulty overcoming these toxic judgments whenever they are unable to differentiate friends from imposters who want to use them rather than develop true friendship and mutuality. The foregoing demonstrates that ASD affects more than the patient. It is a stone cast into the water whose ripples spread in all directions to reach many people including family and friends, subjects of the next chapter.

REFERENCES

Adams, Susan. 2010. "Working with Someone with Asperger's." *Forbes*. August 3. https://www.forbes.com/2010/08/03/asperger-syndrome-workplace-leadership-careers-autism.

Anderson, Connie. 2010. "IAN Research Report #14—April: Grandparents of Children with ASD, Part 1." Interactive Autism Network. https://iancommunity.org/cs/ian_research_reports/ian_research_report_apr_2010.

Autism Speaks. n.d. "Applied Behavior Analysis." https://www.autismspeaks.org/what-autism/treatment/applied-behavior-analysis-aba.

Benson, R. Paul. 2006. "The Impact of Child Symptom Severity on Depressed Mood Among Parents of Children with ASD: The Mediating Role of Stress

Proliferation." *Journal of Autism and Developmental Disorders* 36, no. 5 (July): 685–695.

Bishop, Summer L., Jennifer Richler, C. Albert Cain, and Catherine Lord. 2007. "Predictors of Perceived Negative Impact in Mothers of Children with Autism Spectrum Disorder." *American Journal on Mental Retardation* 6, vol. 112 (November): 450–461.

Boucher, Cheryl, and Kathy Oehler. 2013. *"I Hate to Write!": Tips for Helping Students with Autism Spectrum and Related Disorders Increase Achievement, Meet Academic Standards, and Become Happy, Successful Writers.* Shawnee, KS: AAPC Publishing.

Ewing, Rachel. 2015. "Drexel Releases National Indicators Report on Autism & Adolescent Transitions." *Drexel NOW.* April 21. http://drexel.edu/now /archive/2015/April/Autism-Indicators-Young-Adult-Transition/.

Grandin, Temple. 2017. "Keys to Successful Independent Living, Employment and a Good Social Life for Individuals with Autism and Asperger's." Autism Research Institute, September 26. https://www.autism.com/grandin _independence.

Holtz, Kristen D., Nicole M. Owings, and Amanda K. Ziegert. 2006. *Life Journey through Autism: A Guide for Transition to Adulthood.* Arlington, VA: Organization for Autism Research.

Lasgaard, Mathias, Annette E. Nielsen, Mette Eriksen, and Luc Goossens. 2010. "Loneliness and Social Support in Adolescent Boys with Autism Spectrum Disorders." *Journal of Autism and Developmental Disorders* 40, no. 2 (February): 218–226.

Roux, Anne, Jessica Rast, Julianna Rava, Kristy Anderson, and Paul Shattuck. 2015. "National Indicators Report: Transition into Young Adulthood." Philadelphia: Life Course Outcomes Research Program, A. J. Drexel Autism Institute, Drexel University.

Shattuck, Paul T., Carter Sarah Narendorf, Benjamin Cooper, Paul R. Sterzing, Mary Wagner, and Julie Lounds Taylor. 2012. "Postsecondary Education and Employment among Youth with an Autism Spectrum Disorder." *Pediatrics* 129, no. 6 (June): 1042–1049.

Standifer, Scott. 2009. *Adult Autism and Unemployment: A Guide for Vocational Rehabilitation Professionals.* Columbia: Disability Policy Studies, School of Health Professionals, University of Missouri.

Vicker, Beverly. n.d. "Social Communication and Language Characteristics Associated with High Functioning, Verbal Children and Adults with ASD." Indiana Resource Center for Autism. https://www.iidc.indiana.edu/pages /Social-Communication-and-Language-Characteristics-Associated-with -High-Functioning-Verbal-Children-and-Adults-with-ASD.

Wallis, Lynne. 2012. "Autistic Workers: Loyal, Talented...Ignored." *The Guardian,* April 6. https://www.theguardian.com/money/2012/apr/06/autistic-workers -employers-ignorance.

Woog, Dan. n.d. "Succeeding at Work with Autism." Monster. https://www.monster .com/career-advice/article/succeeding-at-work-with-autism.

7

Effects on Family and Friends

With autism spectrum disorder (ASD), or another disease, disorder, malady, affliction, ailment, or condition, the focus is on patients because they suffer. But a fixation on them risks ignoring family and friends, who likewise anguish over this suffering. Pain is understandable given the range of problems confronting caregivers (whether parents, grandparents, guardians, adoptive parents, or others), including issues that impinge on emotional health, marital relations, sibling dynamics, and the expenses of care. Friends experience their own issues as they toil to interact with a person with ASD given his or her social deficits. Although these problems may seem insurmountable, family and friends may nonetheless feel positive about their kin or comrade, respectively, and in their relations with him or her. Neither are these problems intractable. For example, a new friendship always requires effort at the outset because the two are becoming acquainted. As they come to understand each other, they exert less effort trying to decode nonverbal cues because each knows the other well enough not to need to gauge his or her intentions constantly. Reduced exertions never stagnate into inattentiveness because true friends always make the necessary efforts to help each other in various ways.

FAMILY

Negative Emotional Issues

ASD affects families in a visceral way that may cause emotions to tangle. Diverse emotions prevent their ranking in importance. Angst that stems from ASD's incurability; family members may express frustration that no pill or elixir ends ASD's troubles (Shannon 2011). The problem is acute because they inhabit a world in which vaccination has conquered smallpox and antibiotics can overcome a variety of bacterial infections, but a cure for ASD seems to be a mirage so that the condition appears to be an unjust sentence for an innocent newborn. These sentiments extend to other incurable maladies.

This frustration, perhaps because it is so pernicious, may cause family members to doubt themselves and medical providers. Such frustrations are difficult to detail because of their ubiquity. Amplifying concerns is the fact that medicine, particularly psychiatry, has not always aided families, especially parents (Silberman 2016; Donvan and Zucker 2016). Psychiatry's inadequacy in the early years of autism research is evident in Austrian American physician and ASD pioneer Leo Kanner's refrigerator mom thesis detailed in chapter 2.

Guilt and frustration exacerbate parents' difficulties raising a child with ASD, problems that mount as they struggle to bond with him or her. They may overcompensate by trying to maximize time with him or her in hopes of forming bonds no matter the obstacles. Parents want to hold and cuddle their children; yet a child with ASD who feels discomfort in these settings becomes rigid in rebuffing affection. In the same vein, parents want to bond with their children through making and sustaining eye contact even when such intimacy overwhelms these children, who look at the ground or into space as though fixated on an imaginary spot far from parents' gaze. These dynamics impact sibling relations, a reality examined later in this chapter and in the third case study at the end of this book.

Difficulties multiply when parents cannot console an unhappy child with ASD, so that he or she may erupt in a tantrum, discomforting onlookers, a phenomenon noted in earlier chapters. Such frustration heightens guilt by shaming caregivers. Whether parents, grandparents, guardians, or adoptive parents, caregivers may feel shame at resenting the difficulties of caring for a person with ASD, according to Joyce Shannon's edited book and other literature mentioned earlier. Researchers have long detailed the stresses of caring for a disabled person. Recent findings go beyond these observations to demonstrate that caring for a child with ASD is more difficult than raising someone with another disability (Schwarz 2009). This research emphasizes ASD's special burdens. Because caregivers face strenuous demands, they are at least partly isolated from those whose children have other maladies. In other words, the parents, grandparents, guardians, or adoptive parents of a child with ASD experience social isolation to an uncommon degree. Isolation is difficult to overcome and is a hallmark of ASD, at least as it affects caregivers.

Positive Emotional Issues

Treacherous though ASD's emotional landscape is, caregivers may experience positive moments even when such instances do not lead to euphoria. Nonetheless, caregivers take pride in children's improvements, no matter how small, according to "Autism Spectrum Disorder (ASD)" available online from the Centers for Disease Control and Prevention (CDC) in Atlanta, Georgia. Improvements, when multiplied over time, yield substantial progress. Recall that improvements never cure what is now incurable, but a taciturn child with ASD who struggles with language may, through efforts from caregivers, teachers, language pathologists, and other experts, mature into an adult who can communicate well enough to hold a stable job and live independently (Grandin 2017).

Chapter 2 notes that people once labeled with Asperger's syndrome have a range of interests that they enjoy communicating to others. Their caregivers take pride in nurturing such interests. Many people with ASD, not just those once categorized as having Asperger's syndrome, have interests that may be reinforced through attentive parenting. By strengthening these interests, caregivers may bond with a child with ASD, even one who struggles to make and sustain eye contact or dislikes being held and cuddled. Attention to cues from a child avoids overwhelming him or her with strident emotions so that parents learn to go at his or her emotional tempo.

Moving outside their roles as caregivers, parents may attend support groups to learn and practice new parenting skills, notes the previously mentioned article "Family Support" from the Organization for Autism Research. Support groups offer more than skills by comforting attendees who share the reality of caring for a child with ASD. This camaraderie is evident among military veterans, being marked in those who served in combat. Shared experiences are the basis for common emotional bonds and unity.

Forming these relationships, caregivers may become advocates for their children and for the larger issue of ASD (Autism Speaks n.d.). These efforts raise ASD awareness and heighten public outreach and understanding. A February 2018 Google search with the phrase "autism advocacy groups" yielded nearly 6.2 million websites. Perhaps the most prominent group is Autism Speaks, founded in February 2005 by Robert and Suzanne Wright, the grandparents of a child with ASD. They set out to organize a forum that seeks the best care for people with ASD and that aims to form bonds among caregivers. With $25 million in grants, Autism Speaks has grown into a worldwide ASD advocate that promotes research into ASD's causes, diagnosis of all children with ASD before age two, improvements in treatment and access to the best care, support for children with ASD and their caregivers, and promotion of efforts to help children with ASD grow into adults capable of independent living and work in hopes of improving quality of life and eventually curing the disorder. Autism Speaks envisions a public–private partnership to advance ASD research and treatments. To promote these agendas, Autism Speaks has subsidiaries collectively known as Autism Speaks U. Functioning as an informal online university, it unites teachers, students, and graduates to promote ASD awareness and raise money for research. Pennsylvania State University in University Park formed the first chapter in 2006. Within two years a network of chapters spread to colleges and universities throughout the United States. Through them and by pursuing other avenues, Autism Speaks promotes its aims in local, state and national politics.

EFFECTS ON MARRIAGE

In shaping families, ASD influences marital dynamics because parents, grandparents, guardians, adoptive parents, or other caregivers relate not just to a child with ASD but also to one another. Accordingly, ASD raises several issues including possible financial instability, a concern echoed in an April 2016 article "A Meta-Synthesis on Parenting a Child with Autism" available online from the National Center for Biotechnology Information referenced in earlier chapters. Financial difficulties are sensitive and pervasive, meriting a section later in this chapter.

The emphasis here is on noneconomic issues, the first being the imperative that parents become knowledgeable about the medicines they administer to a child with ASD. Chapter 5 discusses several medicines, noting the need to tailor them to an ASD person's circumstances. The National Institute of Mental Health (NIMH), referenced in previous chapters, recommends that parents complete six months' training to ensure their acquisition of skills necessary to maximize a child with ASD's quality of life through proper medication and behavioral modification. Important is parents' recognition that medicines alone, no matter their combination and dosage, can achieve only partial improvements (American Academy of Child and Adolescent Psychiatry 2016). As noted earlier, this recognition may be tardy in a world where modern medicine offers vaccines, antibiotics, and other agents to eliminate some infectious diseases in some parts of the globe. Along these lines, the accent must be on parental attempts to minimize ASD children's unpleasant behaviors by reducing tantrums, aggression, self injury, and other counterproductive behaviors mentioned in chapter 4 and to amplify sociable behaviors. These efforts unite parents, grandparents, guardians, adoptive parents, or other caregivers in the shared goal of optimizing their child's quality of life. Whenever caretakers disagree on the best approach, the marriage suffers, stress mounts, and husband and wife find themselves embroiled in arguments (Bluth et al. 2013).

Second, parents, grandparents, guardians, adoptive parents, or other caregivers must plan and participate in their child's education. The immediate issue is likely to be whether to put a child with ASD in classes that provides the least restrictive environment (known as mainstreaming) or in special education. Tension builds no matter the decision and is acute when husband and wife disagree. Before reaching a decision, caretakers must assess the credentials of those available to evaluate their child. An evaluator's decision to favor either special education or immersion in regular classes is not binding whenever parents disagree with the findings and request an opinion from an outside expert in a process known as an independent educational evaluation (IEE) (PACER Center n.d.). When a professional deems a child with ASD eligible for special education and the caretakers agree, the school creates an individualized education program (IEP). This step draws on information from parents or other caregivers, teachers, administrators, school counselors, and other professionals in accordance with state laws. Note that because education is a local and state matter, no federal guidelines exist to regulate or unify the contents of IEPs, even though the federal government plays a role in education. The nature of federalism in the United States requires, with few exceptions, that the federal role in education be secondary to local and state preferences. (Countervailing examples, like the federal decision to integrate Little Rock High School in Little Rock, Arkansas in 1954 despite local and state opposition, may cause erroneous perceptions that the federal government always dictates what schools can and cannot do. This assumption follows from intense media coverage of divisive educational issues that amplify marginal viewpoints over the consensus.)

Returning to ASD and other disability issues, the determination that a child with ASD requires an IEP acknowledges, tacitly or overtly, that he or she is disabled. The decision that he or she has a disability likely does not shock parents because physicians and perhaps social workers have already paved the way for this conclusion. Nevertheless confirmation of disability heightens tensions in couples that are already struggling to care for a child or children with ASD. Moreover, at every juncture in the process of evaluation and remediation, parents who disagree over the best course of action for an ASD child or children grow tenser. Finally, the steps that determine a child with ASD's status, if taken at a public school, occur at its expense not a family's. In other words, taxpayers become the payee in lieu of the family.

Third, caretakers, perhaps trained according to NIMH guidelines referenced earlier, aim to modify the behavior of a child with ASD through positive reinforcement (a reward for good behavior). But such reinforcement sometimes fails, exasperating parents and stressing their marriage. Even a reward that works weakens when children with ASD lose interest in it. These instances nevertheless yield options. NIMH guidelines urge caregivers to shorten the interval between good performance and positive reinforcement because prompt reward has the best chance of capturing and sustaining the attention of children with ASD. But promptness can be difficult to achieve when school performance is at stake. Children with ASD who excel on a math quiz, for example, forget this achievement when they must wait until returning home for a reward, dooming what parents had intended as prompt positive feedback, further stressing their marriage. These circumstances may push parents into the trap of overusing a reward to compensate for its delay. Overuse is no better than any other attempt to overcompensate, and parents again feel marital tensions. Even when it works, a child with ASD may outgrow a reward so that what worked in childhood becomes tedious rather than interesting in adolescence. These frustrations stress marriages even when couples work to unify their goals and methods.

Fourth, the need for constant care of a child with ASD can strain a couple's sex lives (Aylaz, Tilmaz, and Polat 2012). The coauthors could gather data from only a narrow range of participants because most Turkish parents are uncomfortable discussing their sex lives. The taboo surrounding such discussions prevented participating parents from publicizing their views so that none was willing to have his or her voice recorded when they answered researchers' questions. With the data they had, the coauthors conclude that the primary burden of caring for a child with ASD falls on the mother. Resenting this unfairness, she withholds sex from her husband, leading him to feel sexually unfulfilled and deprived. These tensions are evident to anyone who has experienced such deprivation.

Fifth, ASD's effects on divorce rates have concerned researchers since 1943, when Austrian American physician and autism pioneer Leo Kanner scrutinized the parents of the first 11 children with ASD he treated. Kanner rated three of the marriages "dismal failures," and even the strongest unions were "cold and formal" (Serris 2017). These criticisms persist in research asserting that 80 percent of marriages in which at least one child has ASD end in divorce, and the issue remains contentious with four studies published between 2004 and 2015 tabulating different divorce rates in various parts of the world. In the largest study to date (Brewington 2010), scientists queried 78,000 parents in the United States, with 913 having one or more children with ASD. The study found that the divorce rate among parents of children with ASD mirrors that of parents of neurotypical children, implying that the first set of parents has no more stress than the second. The study suggests that divorce rates are identical because the parents of children with ASD cannot afford to divorce, bond more rather than less tightly in response to their social isolation, or are older than many other parents and so have had years or even decades to build a strong marriage. Because roughly half of all marriages in the United States end in divorce, the rate among parents of children with ASD cannot be the 80 percent claimed in other studies.

Another study surveyed 500 parents. Researchers noted that mothers participated in larger numbers than fathers, a circumstance common in such surveys. Questions were open ended to permit narrative answers. One mother admitted that caring for a child with ASD put enormous "strain on the marriage." Other mothers regretted a lack of quality time with their husbands, who disbelieved that their child had ASD despite a doctor's diagnosis. Judging from the results, couples' tempers were short, some fathers avoided coming home at day's end and were unwilling to face the reality of ASD, marriages no longer seemed normal, and couples struggled to give a child with ASD constant attention.

Not all responses were negative. Some parents affirmed that a child's ASD diagnosis strengthened their marriage as they united against a common foe. Other couples stated that ASD taught them the true meaning of "unconditional love" (Serris 2017) and that this love unified them despite adversity. One husband noted how strong his marriage had become since an ASD diagnosis in his and his wife's child. Another husband and father encapsulated these dynamics, saying that the reality of ASD either cements or weakens unions.

EFFECTS ON GRANDPARENTS

In April 2010 a new study (Kennedy Krieger Institute 2010) showed that of the more than 2,600 grandparents queried, nearly one-third had been the first to raise concerns about grandchildren's development, and another 49 percent had supported their children (first filial generation) in seeking a doctor's evaluation of children (second filial generation). For clarity, the first filial generation consisted of neurotypical adults (the parents of the second filial generation) whereas the second filial generation consisted of children suspected of having ASD. Almost 90 percent of these grandparents reported that the ordeal of ASD brought them closer to their grandchildren. These same grandparents nonetheless fretted that their neurotypical children, raising children with ASD of their own, had too much stress. Nonetheless, 92 percent of grandparents surveyed believed that their marriage had strengthened to combat ASD's intrusion in their lives and in their neurotypical children and ASD grandchildren's lives. These grandparents reported support from their spouses throughout ASD's travails. Roughly 15 percent of grandparents had at least two grandchildren with ASD, strengthening the conviction that faulty genes cause ASD even when the environment modifies the severity. Some two-thirds of these grandchildren were siblings and the rest cousins.

Of grandparents surveyed, almost all interacted frequently with an ASD grandchild. Roughly 10 percent lived with him or her, as had been true years earlier, and another 46 percent resided less than 25 miles away. Nearly 15 percent had moved closer to their grandchildren in hopes of better nurturing them. Another 7 percent had moved into their grandchildren's homes to help them upon learning of an ASD diagnosis. Grandparents' opinions were important enough that 71 percent were consulted about their grandchildren's medical needs. More than 15 percent shuttled their grandchildren to and from school and medical appointments at least weekly. Another 31 percent cared for grandchildren at least weekly when other daycare was unavailable.

Such grandparents are rarely idle. Ninety-nine percent researched ASD's signs and symptoms in hopes of better understanding and nurturing their afflicted grandchildren. Grandparents' activism spread into other areas, with almost half participating in walks and fundraisers for ASD research. One-third contacted local, state, and federal representatives to request more money for ASD research for causes and treatments. Slightly fewer (31 percent) took the extra step of attending ASD conferences or workshops to increase their knowledge about causes and treatments. Their financial burdens receive coverage later.

EFFECTS ON SIBLINGS

Neurotypical siblings, too, feel ASD's effects. Sibling dynamics are difficult to summarize given their dependence on several factors. For example, the greater the strain on marriages, the worse are relations among siblings (Rivers and Stoneman 2003). Curiously, parents who underwent intensive marriage counseling had children whose sibling rivalries were more detrimental than was true of parents who sought less marital counseling. But not all data are negative. Even when parents believe that children's sibling rivalries are harmful, siblings reported positive relationships among one another, and overall most reported good rapport throughout the family. Where extended family, friends, and neighbors offered parents and their child or children with ASD strong support, siblings had good relations. Yet support was less effective with siblings on uneasy terms, a circumstance that also applies to neurotypical siblings.

Siblings of a high functioning child with ASD tend to have poorer relationships than siblings of neurotypical children. These difficulties, conspicuous in siblings between ages 6 and 11, may mar other aspects of life. For example, siblings may mimic a high functioning ASD brother or sister by misbehaving in school even when they describe their lives as carefree. Sisters from ages 12 to 16 (one high functioning and the other neurotypical) had the best self esteem. Brothers and sisters (again in roughly 1:1 ratios between high functioning and neurotypical) with the best self esteem were the most socially adept whereas those with the worst self-image had the least social skills. Finally, neurotypical siblings who thought well of themselves applauded their parents' care of a high functioning child with ASD. The converse was also true (Rivers and Stoneman 2003).

Children with ASD demand constant care, leaving parents few opportunities to nurture their other children (Autism Society n.d.). Even the most responsible parents, willing to sacrifice their own happiness for their ASD child's welfare, often lack the energy and time to make the same sacrifices for their neurotypical children, a circumstance that exacerbates sibling rivalries. Factors include embarrassment at an ASD sibling's misbehavior (especially in public), resentment at parents for spending so much time with him, exasperation at his poor interactions with them, fear that his outbursts may endanger them, fatigue at the continual demands of compensating for his misbehavior, concern over parents' mental and physical well being, and uncertainty about the future and their role in supporting him.

Given these circumstances and common sense, parents reassure their neurotypical children. Parents should tell these children that a brother or sister has ASD, describing its signs and symptoms in as much detail as is age appropriate and as early as practicable. Simple language and concepts are best for young siblings whereas adolescents may be ready to discuss ASD's probable genetic causes, though such information cannot hope to be comprehensive, especially because scientists and medical experts do not have a complete understanding of ASD's genetic roots. Parents must be mindful of issues that concern siblings. Young siblings typically want to know how to respond to their ASD brother or sister's outbursts, whereas older ones usually want to know what to tell their friends about ASD. In addition, adolescents often want to know the future course of treatment and their role in helping him or her.

FAMILY FINANCES

Detrimental to any marriage, financial problems threaten many families including those with one or more children with ASD. The demands, financial and otherwise, of caring for people with ASD extends from birth to death (Holtz, Owings, and Ziegert 2006). As they age, these demands intensify because they are likely to outlive parents, who must amass assets for care past their deaths. Financial planning has several goals including establishment, where possible, of a trust to insulate an ASD son or daughter from financial peril. Other vehicles for amassing resources include an Individual Retirement Account (IRA), a 401 (k), real estate, equity in the home (which ideally is owned free and clear), life insurance, and other financial instruments. Disability payments are straightforward, not an investment issue, and may also be part of the mix. The details of investment options may require parents to consult an accountant, attorney, financial planner, or another expert specializing in these areas.

Not all families can marshal enough resources to care for a child with ASD from cradle to grave even with regular disability payments or other government assistance. Financial problems loom large because raising a child with ASD (adults excluded from this analysis) costs between $1.4 and $2.4 million (Buescher et al. 2014). The high range of this estimate applies to families of mentally deficient children with ASD. Without such impairment, costs tend to reduce toward the lower figure. In total, U.S. families spend $61 billion annually to care for children with ASD, whereas UK families spend $4.5 billion. The disparity between these numbers stems from the fact that the United States has more children with ASD as a consequence of having a larger population and higher per person medical costs than the United Kingdom. Numerous studies indicate that the United States has among the world's highest medical costs per capita with disappointing results given lackluster longevity averages. Neither U.S. nor UK data estimate the costs of caring for adults with ASD, an omission acknowledged earlier. The expenses of raising children with ASD in the United States or United Kingdom derive principally from special education, where public schools are not the sole component, and lost parental income. For adults with ASD, costs mount when they live in institutions or cannot work. In his June 2014 interview with Autism Speaks, David Mandell, physician and director of the Center for Mental Health Policy and Services Research at the University of Pennsylvania in Philadelphia, acknowledges these costs as the best outcome because the expense of caring for a person with ASD averts the accumulating costs of neglect. In brief, the earlier a person with ASD receives care, the less expensive it is over the long term (Roux and Shattuck 2014).

Grandparents of ASD grandchildren often shoulder a financial burden (Kennedy Krieger Institute 2010). Of grandparents surveyed, 22 percent diverted money from buying something they wanted to pay part of their ASD grandchild's costs of care. Eighteen percent were the primary caregivers while their children (the parents of the child with ASD) worked.

Eleven percent sacrificed their future stability by draining retirement accounts or borrowing money. Almost three fifths worked more hours or took a second job to devote more money to their ASD grandchild's care. Some spent more than $500 per month on his or her care, though the majority spent less.

EFFECTS ON FRIENDS

Although many people with ASD have few social skills, most want friends. Individuals with ASD who desire friends develop social skills early in life. Friendships may insulate them from bullying in school as children and on the job as adults. These realities require friends of a person with ASD to become knowledgeable about ASD so they can reassure others who are unsure whether or how to interact with him or her. In this way, ASD challenges neurotypical friends to advocate for him or her and by extension for greater knowledge, respect, and compassion for all people with ASD. That is, ASD expands friends' horizons and abilities to differentiate between what is important in life and what is trivial and transitory. The closer the neurotypical friend, the more likely he or she is to defend people with ASD from insults, prejudices, preconceptions, or misunderstandings.

ASD teaches neurotypical friends patience because people with ASD form friendships slowly, according to the Autism Society article referenced above. Given the strong interests of people with ASD, particularly those without cognitive impairments, ASD challenges a neurotypical friend to expand his or her curiosity and worldview by listening to descriptions of their interests. These friendships require generosity with time because interests may be described at length. Moreover, ASD prompts neurotypical friends to become good communicators because people with ASD may not be adept at sharing and processing information, especially in cases of cognitive impairment.

CONCLUSION

ASD affects family and friends in multiple ways, stirring turbulent emotions, both negative and positive. ASD tests marriages by pulling parents in several directions at once. They advocate for a child with ASD by seeking the best education, intensifying care by managing medicines, modifying behaviors, and building the resources to achieve financial security from birth to death. Parents are tested in other ways because the demands of care may diminish their sex lives, drain emotions and finances, precipitate arguments, heighten stress, and lead to divorce. Yet all is not doom

and gloom because some marriages strengthen as couples unite in pursuing the best outcome for their child with ASD. ASD also affects grandparents, many of whom care for a grandchild with ASD under a variety of
circumstances. Some grandparents contribute money to this care, thereby
sacrificing future comfort. Siblings respond in many ways to their ASD
brother or sister and to concurrent family dynamics. Moreover, ASD challenges friends of a person with ASD to grow in knowledge, compassion,
sensitivity, and other attributes. The next chapter turns from these issues
to prevention, a hypothetical subject because scientists and medical
experts do not understand how to avert a disorder present at life's beginning and under genetic control at a time when gene therapy is emergent.

REFERENCES

American Academy of Child and Adolescent Psychiatry. 2016. "Autism
    Spectrum Disorder: Parents' Medication Guide." Washington, DC.
    https://www.aacap.org/App_Themes/AACAP/Docs/resource
    _centers/autism/Autism_Spectrum_Disorder_Parents_Medication
    _Guide.pdf.
Autism Society. n.d. "Siblings." http://www.autism-society.org/living-with
    -autism/family-issues/siblings/.
Autism Speaks. n.d. "Special Education and Advocacy." https://www
    .autismspeaks.org/family-services/community-connections/special
    -education-and-advocacy.
Aylaz, Rukuye, Ulviye Tilmaz, and Sevinc Polat. 2012. "Effect of Difficul-
    ties Experienced by Parents of Autistic Children on Their Sexual
    Life: A Qualitative Study." *Sexuality and Disability* 30, no. 4
    (December): 395–406.
Bluth, Karen, Patricia N. E. Roberson, Rhett M. Billen, and Juli M. Sams.
    2013. "A Stress Model for Couples Parenting Children with Autism
    Spectrum Disorders and the Introduction of a Mindfulness Inter-
    vention." *Journal of Family Review* 5, no. 2 (September): 194–213.
Brewington, Kelly. 2010. "Autism in Kids Doesn't Drive Parents to Divorce."
    May 20, *Baltimore Sun.* http://www.baltimoresun.com/bs-mtblog
    -2010-05-autism_divorce_rate_myth-story.html.
Buescher, A. V., Z. Cidav, M. Knapp, and D. S. Mandell. 2014. "Costs of
    Autism Spectrum Disorders in the United Kingdom and the United
    States." *Journal of the American Medical Association Pediatrics*
    168, no. 8 (August): 721–728.
Donvan, John, and Caren Zucker. 2016. *In a Different Key: The Story of
    Autism.* New York: Crown.
Grandin, Temple. 2017. "Keys to Successful Independent Living, Employ-
    ment and a Good Social Life for Individuals with Autism and

Asperger's." Autism Research Institute, September 26. https://www.autism.com/grandin_independence.

Holtz, Kristen D., Nicole M. Owings, and Amanda K. Ziegert. 2006. *Life Journey through Autism: A Guide for Transition to Adulthood.* Arlington, VA: Organization for Autism Research.

Kennedy Krieger Institute. 2010. "New Survey Finds Grandparents Play Key Role in the Lives of Children with Autism." April 6. https://www.kennedykrieger.org/overview/news/new-survey-finds-grandparents-play-key-role-lives-children-autism.

PACER Center. n.d. "Understanding the Special Education Process." http://www.pacer.org/parent/resources/understanding-the-spec-ed-process.asp.

Rivers, Jessica Wood, and Zolinda Stoneman. 2003. "Sibling Relationships When a Child Has Autism: Marital Stress and Support Coping." *Journal of Autism and Development Disorders* 33, no. 4 (August): 383–394.

Roux, Anne, and Paul T. Shattuck. 2014. "Autism: Moving toward an Innovation and Investment Mindset." *Journal of the American Medical Association Pediatrics* 168, no. 8 (August): 698–699.

Schwarz, Joel. 2009. "Mothers of Children with Autism Have Higher Parental Stress, Psychological Distress." *University of Washington News,* July 8.

Serris, Marina. 2017. "Under a Looking Glass: What's the Truth about Autism and Marriage?" *Interactive Autism Network,* April 11. https://iancommunity.org/whats-truth-about-autism-and-marriage.

Shannon, Joyce Brennfleck. 2011. *Autism and Pervasive Developmental Disorders Sourcebook.* 2nd ed. Detroit: Omnigraphics.

Silberman, Steve. 2016. *The Legacy of Autism and the Future of Neurodiversity.* New York: Avery.

8

Prevention

In the case of autism spectrum disorder (ASD), prevention strategies are uncertain at least partly because scientists and medical experts have not pinpointed the causes to everyone's satisfaction, though faulty genes must play the chief role. Without identifying every dysfunctional gene, medical practitioners cannot hope to silence them, thereby preventing most if not all ASD signs and symptoms. Even supposing these genes were known, gene therapy is not advanced enough to disable them. In the absence of foolproof strategies of prevention, people with ASD may still have options, however limited, many centered on diet and other common-sense measures. Even if their effects on ASD are small, they remain sound options for maintaining robust health. For example, the directive to consume sufficient vitamins, minerals, and other nutrients from the best, freshest foods is sensible for everyone in all walks of life.

A VARIETY OF STRATEGIES

Scientists, physicians, nutritionists, and other professionals have long debated whether and the degree to which ASD is preventable. The consensus is that ASD is not understood well enough to guarantee prevention in the way that isolation prevents infectious disease transmissions. Medical professionals have not identified ASD's causes with complete precision, though the principal research agencies point the finger at harmful genes (National Institutes of Health 2005, 2008). These overviews corroborate Chapter 3's summary of recent thinking about ASD's causes, highlighting the role of genes.

To the degree that experts continue to debate causes, uncertainty about them translates into the absence of ironclad directives for preventing ASD, meaning that prevention strategies may involve some guesswork. Strategies exist, and are worth pursuing for overall benefits to the body if not always for preventing ASD. While some websites tout preventive strategies, they often fail to cite peer reviewed literature.

People with ASD labor to minimize social deficits, usually with help from parents and professionals even though minimization can never prevent any ASD sign or symptom. Other examples abound, but the difficulty lies in how best to minimize signs and symptoms. Interventions for social inadequacies include applied behavior analysis therapy (ABA), augmentative and alternative communication, pharmacology, psychotherapy, dietary manipulations, sensory integration therapy, and social skills training (Tweed, Connolly, and Beaulieu 2009). The breadth of ASD's signs and symptoms means that no therapy suits all patients.

DIET AND EXPECTANT MOTHERS

Alcohol

Expectant mothers want to deliver the healthiest newborns. Advice for them comes from all quarters and cannot receive full treatment here. Much of it is general and applies to all pregnant women, not just those at risk for bearing a baby with ASD. Advice may be grouped in broad categories like diet and nutrition. Within this category are numerous directives for preventing ASD, including the reduction or elimination of alcohol and caffeine. Alcohol deserves scrutiny because its toxicity is evident in the fact that people have died or shortened their lives by drinking too much too often, but even moderate amounts may be unhealthy. In expectant mothers at risk for having a baby with ASD, alcohol appears to be an uncertain factor (Eliasen et al. 2010). Expectant mothers who drink some alcohol but not inordinate amounts seem not to be at heightened risk of delivering an autistic baby, but those who binge drink even once during pregnancy have a slightly elevated risk of having a newborn with ASD. Limited alcohol consumption likely poses negligible risk to pregnant women in danger of bearing an ASD baby but nonetheless, they are advised to avoid alcohol because it undermines the fetus' health (Singer et al. 2017).

On the other hand, a gene (likely multiple genes) may predispose someone to having both ASD and alcoholism, though the relevant research has yet to receive full scrutiny. A family with at least one member with ASD is likely to be at greater risk that some family member, the person with ASD or another, will be an alcoholic than any member of a family without ASD. Under such circumstances the responsible person, either with ASD or related to someone who has it, avoids alcohol. Other studies conclude that expectant mothers who drink too much alcohol are in danger of delivering a baby with ASD, but this finding is not the scientific and medical consensus. Moreover, schoolchildren with ASD are at risk of alcoholism because their difficulties interacting with peers may lead them to cope by drinking alcohol. The same rationale applies to the risk of drug addiction. Use of alcohol or drugs or both to mask suffering has long been practiced worldwide, making ASD no anomaly. Given these dangers, recommendations suggest that people with ASD restrict or eliminate alcohol as follows: women should drink no more than a glass of alcohol per day, men less than age 65 may consume as many as two glasses per day whereas those over 65 should not exceed one glass, and anyone unable to regulate consumption should never drink alcohol.

Vitamin and Mineral Supplements

Although the practice of supplementing the diet with minerals was a goal of human and livestock nutrition in the nineteenth century, little was accomplished before the 1912 discovery of the first vitamin (vitamin A). The attention lavished on this breakthrough included the 1929 Nobel Prize in physiology or medicine for the discoverer and the development of a vitamin and mineral supplement industry, especially in the United States. Given these circumstances and bringing our coverage to the present, attention focuses on the role of these supplements in preventing several maladies including ASD. By definition a vitamin is a compound vital to health, and minerals also cannot be neglected. It follows that optimal health requires ingestion of all vitamins and minerals in proper amounts. Over supplementation may injure the body when it stores excess nutrients in fat or be harmless when excreted. Yet the media, as has long been true, are sometimes less interested in an even-handed treatment of all nutrients than in focusing on those whose popularity is increasing.

For example, vitamin D, sometimes known as the sunshine vitamin, is in the news; a reasonable approach given its shortage in many people. The body can acquire it in two ways. One is to expose the skin to sunlight, which the body uses to synthesize the vitamin. The other is through supplementation, whether in tablets or in fortified foods given that few foods aside from fatty fish naturally have much vitamin D. The issue may pivot more on lessening signs and symptoms than on preventing ASD. In 2008, the nonprofit Vitamin D Council in San Luis Obispo, California, conducted perhaps the most ambitious study of the relationship between ASD and vitamin D, finding that ASD afflicted more people where clouds were numerous, or air pollution was noticeable, by minimizing sunlight. Moreover, the darker the skin, the greater is the risk of ASD because dark skin screens out the sunlight necessary for manufacturing vitamin D. These findings demonstrate that vitamin D lessens ASD signs and symptoms and hint that it may have a preventative role. Prevention would require researchers to prove that no pregnant woman at risk of delivering a newborn with ASD does so when she acquires sufficient vitamin D. Proof is difficult to achieve whenever reasoning, such as that applied to ASD and vitamin D, depends on induction. Pregnant women who do not consume enough of the vitamin risk having a baby with ASD, again suggesting rather than proving a preventive role for vitamin D (Vinkhuyzen et al. 2017). Newborns with the least vitamin D are most likely to be born with ASD, strengthening the link between ASD and vitamin D because a newborn can only have gotten vitamin D from the mother; but again, the conclusion rests on probability rather than certainty.

A circumstantial case can be made that a number of vitamins, minerals, and other nutrients may prevent ASD. First, returning to vitamin D, children with ASD are likely deficient and so suffer from constipation, diarrhea, and gastrointestinal problems as a result. They tend not to eat a variety of foods, lessening opportunities for ingesting vitamin D, though recall that few foods have much of it. Second, some medical practitioners advise children with ASD to take supplements with large amounts of vitamins and minerals in order to exceed the recommended daily allowance (RDA) of these nutrients. At high levels of supplementation, the practice is known as mega dosing. Third, the Vinkhuyzen article remarks that vitamins A, C, and B6 (pyridoxine), the mineral magnesium, omega 3 fatty acids (the type of fats in fish), and dimethylglycine (an amino acid abbreviated DMG and thought to strengthen the immune system), improve the health of children with ASD. Several lines of research recommend vitamin B9 (folic acid or folate) consumption in hopes of lessening ASD signs and symptoms or possibly preventing it. Nonetheless, research dismisses many of these recommendations, including mega doses of vitamins C and B6 and inclusion of omega 3 fatty acids in the diet, as irrelevant to ASD's treatment, let alone prevention. Elimination of gluten or dairy from the diet is equally unhelpful.

Enhanced Water

The availability of bottled water in stores and the belief that it is somehow more healthful than tap water lead the public to wonder whether it has any medicinal properties. Along these lines is an inquiry into whether it might prevent ASD. This water goes by many names and is derived from a variety of sources and preparatory techniques. For simplicity this chapter refers to it as enhanced water in accord with the public's conviction that it must be superior to justify the price. Sellers like APEC Water Systems in City of Industry, California, assert that children with ASD should drink enhanced water, but such claims do not prove prevention and are not credible coming from companies motivated by profit. Little distinguishes enhanced water from any other type of water. The difference comes down to personal preference rather than scientific evidence. Even the International Bottled Water Association, which bills itself the "authoritative source of information about all types of bottled water," defends enhanced water's healthfulness only in the weakest way. It notes that enhanced water has no calories, sugar, caffeine, or artificial colors or flavors. Yet tap water has exactly these traits, leaving nothing to differentiate the two. A February 2018 Google search yielded no peer reviewed publications about the relationship between consumption of enhanced water and ASD. For these reasons, no proof exists that enhanced water, despite its popularity, is innately healthful let alone prevents ASD.

Probiotics

Like vitamin D, probiotics (beneficial bacteria and yeasts) are a hot topic. The article "What Can Be Done to Prevent Autism Now?" (McDonnell 2010) tells expectant mothers to ingest "high quality probiotics" to prevent ASD in a newborn (McDonnell, 2010). Again, no evidence accompanies the article, though probiotics benefit the gastrointestinal system and so likely aid people with ASD who suffer gastrointestinal problems. Under these circumstances, probiotics probably lessen at least some ASD signs and symptoms, whether in newborn, child, adolescent, or adult. This line of reasoning, promising though it may be, is a hunch. Pregnant women who ingest probiotics may prevent ASD in their babies, but the reasoning is convoluted and circumstantial (Velasquez-Manoff 2012). The bacterium *Lactobacillus reuteri* appears to lessen in mice behaviors that would in humans be ASD signs and symptoms (Buffington et al. 2016). Of course, mice are not humans, and even if the findings are accurate and apply to humans, proof remains elusive that any probiotic or combination prevents ASD.

Organic Foods

Another popular topic is organic foods and organic farming. The two appear to promise a return to a golden age when synthetic chemicals did not endanger people and the environment. This nostalgia supposes that the consumption of organic foods can prevent, improve, or cure myriad ailments. For simplicity, an organic food is one that must be free from synthetic chemicals, that cannot have been derived through genetic engineering, and that must have been produced on a farm that eschews these supposed dangers. This book does not participate in the tumult over genetically engineered or genetically modified (abbreviated GE or GM) plants, animals, or foods except to note that no crop, livestock, or food derived from agriculture is free from genetic modification. The process of domestication in prehistory modified plants and animal genetics. These changes have accelerated since then.

Our concern is whether organic foods, thought to be especially wholesome, might prevent ASD. Expectant mothers are told to eat organic foods, especially organic green leafy vegetables, to prevent ASD in their newborns. But these articles cobble together a string of assertions without evidence of prevention, though green leafy vegetables, organic or not, have many nutrients and benefit anyone who includes them in the diet.

Sucrose

Another issue is ingestion of the sugar sucrose, found in quantity in sugarcane stalks and the sugar beet taproot. Other sugars are abundant in the biota but cannot receive treatment here. In its derivation, sugar (sucrose) is as natural as any other food but is the archetypal nutritional outcast because it has no nutrients—no protein, vitamins, minerals, antioxidants—nothing of any value except calories, which are too plentiful in the developed world to have real value. Multiple lines of research recommend reductions in sucrose consumption. Too much sugar may damage the brain's D2 receptors, thereby impairing attention and learning, an injury that may intensify emotional outbursts and impulses (Volknow et al. 2009). If sugar ingestion causes aspects of attention deficit and hyperactivity disorder (ADHD), then this research should extend to ASD if the two are related. To be sure, ASD and ADHD share signs and symptoms, but this overlap does not necessitate their unification as the same disorder. Part of the problem is that pediatricians tend to diagnose a child with ADHD and only later change the diagnosis to ASD because the two are so similar. In sum, conflation of ADHD and ASD is never warranted, weakening attempts to make sugar an ASD cause and its elimination an ASD prevention. ASD prevention aside, pregnant women and everyone else, should reduce or eliminate sugar to maintain or improve health and to ensure the best outcome for their child.

A wholesome, nutritious diet is recommended for people with ASD (Ansel 2018), advice that applies to everyone so that no special value may accrue to those with ASD. In addition, no connection between such a diet and ASD prevention, an issue separate from lessening signs and symptoms, is justifiable. A good diet benefits people with ASD but may not prevent ASD.

TOXINS

Many studies confirm the dangers of pesticides, dyes, and other synthetic chemicals to people with ASD. The most damning research links pesticide exposure in pregnant women to the delivery of newborns with ASD, demonstrating that pesticides may contribute to ASD onset and severity in a fetus and implying that their avoidance may prevent ASD. Two studies suffice in a chapter that cannot treat all. In the first, a fetus' risk of developing ASD was strongest during the mother's second and third trimesters for those who lived near farms where pesticides are regularly applied (Shelton et al. 2014). In the second, links were made between ASD and the spraying of pesticides to kill mosquitoes, an important effort given the dangers of mosquito borne diseases. Zika virus and the *Aedes aegypti* mosquito that transmits it have repeatedly made recent news (Sifferlin 2016). Because pesticides are thought to damage the brain's neurotransmitters, these chemicals might cause or contribute to ASD, which is a neurological condition. But this damage, when it occurs before birth, implies that pesticide elimination may prevent the malady. Increasing pesticide use may at least partly explain why more children are diagnosed with ASD every year.

Another toxin is the metal mercury, whose worldwide prevalence heightens concern over its harmfulness. Worries shape debate over a synthetic type of mercury used to preserve vaccines in storage, a practice overlapping with issues in the next chapter. Here the foci are on dental fillings that contain mercury and on mercury contaminated fish in the food supply. Overlap in signs and symptoms of mercury poisoning and of ASD leads to conclusions that mercury causes the disorder.

As for mercury-containing fish, studies acknowledge that mercury may injure children (Oken and Bellinger 2008). Such statements neither prove that mercury causes ASD, nor that the metal's absence prevents it. Although pregnant women are encouraged to limit fish intake, it stops short of linking expectant mothers' consumption of mercury-containing fish to ASD in newborns (Yau et al. 2014).

LIFESTYLE

As a lifestyle choice, exercise benefits people in many ways, leading to the supposition that it might also benefit people with ASD and even prevent ASD. Two factors are in play: expectant mothers' increased body mass correlates with high risk of having a newborn with ASD, and pregnant women's increased weight causes gestational diabetes, which in turn may lead a fetus to develop ASD. Recent peer reviewed studies in *Pediatrics* and the *Journal of the American Medical Association* recommend that pregnant women exercise to prevent gaining too much weight (Moninger n.d.). If this recommendation applies to ASD, then expectant mothers who exercise should minimize ASD in newborns. (Note that this reasoning depends on extrapolation of a finding in one group to another group, and that an unwarranted extrapolation destroys the reasoning, thereby supplying no real information about ASD prevention.)

Numerous studies implicate atmospheric pollution as a cause of ASD, making natural the supposition that an air filter, by cleansing air, might prevent the condition. German air filter manufacturer IQAir (hardly an unbiased source) asserts that atmospheric pollution causes ASD, noting that children living with this pollution and with the MET gene, a faulty variant of a normal gene, are three times more likely to have ASD than children without the allele (IQAir n.d.). This assertion requires that air pollution activates the gene and may be wrong because the study's afflicted children lived amid more air pollution than average children so that pollution may be the lone factor. Nonetheless, because genes are inherited at conception, those with MET, if it is a factor, must be predisposed to ASD before birth irrespective of air quality. With air quality in limbo, IQAir's ASD claims may carry no weight, especially because it has incentives to celebrate research that might yield profits.

Electronic devices, ubiquitous in the modern world, carry health risks. Dunckley (2016) amplifies the association between these devices and ASD, emphasizing that computer and television screens over stimulate children with ASD, a phenomenon she calls "electronic screen syndrome." This syndrome states that electronic devices produce electromagnetic waves (the full spectrum of light, whether visible or not) that overexcite children with ASD. If too much exposure to electromagnetic waves causes or contributes to ASD, then the electronic devices that emit them must be guilty. The absence of these devices and their electromagnetic waves might curtail ASD signs and symptoms, but improvement does not guarantee prevention. The fact that all humans receive at least some exposure to electromagnetic waves weakens an attempt to pinpoint them as ASD's cause and their absence as ASD prevention. As an analogy, all people receive at least some exposure to sunlight; yet the fact that not everyone develops a form of skin cancer weakens an attempt to pinpoint sunlight as the cause of skin cancers. Other factors must be in play such that sunlight's absence cannot prevent all cases of skin cancer.

DRUGS

Like electronic devices, drugs are part of modernity. Perhaps the most ubiquitous is nicotine, being inhaled by smoking tobacco. But not all studies pinpoint nicotine as a cause of ASD (Jung, Lee, McKee, and Picciotto 2017). Uncertainty about nicotine's role in ASD means that not every expectant mother delivers a neurotypical newborn just because she does not smoke. Of course, nicotine's many dangers should dissuade pregnant women from smoking for their own and their newborn's health. These dangers should prompt everybody to avoid nicotine and tobacco smoke, whether direct or secondhand.

Other drugs, really byproducts of microbial action, are the many types of antibiotics. They have spared countless people from death by bacterial infection, but their action in children with ASD is not fully understood. A correlation was found between increases since the 1980s in the use of augmentin, a broad-spectrum antibiotic related to penicillin, and an increase in ASD diagnoses (Fallon 2005). This trend may result from the fact that children below age three who take it have more ammonia, which impairs cognition, in their bodies, though more research is needed to document a role for augmentin in cognitive impairment and a link among augmentin, ammonia, and ASD. Even if an expectant mother can prevent ASD in newborns by eschewing augmentin and possibly other antibiotics, this behavior is counterproductive when she has a dangerous bacterial infection. Antibiotics can change ASD's signs and symptoms in children, though again the mechanism at work is not fully known and changes in signs and symptoms cannot prevent ASD in children who already have it (Benson 2016).

Earlier chapters note the prevalence of depression in children and adults with ASD. A Canadian study linked an elevated risk of bearing a baby with ASD to antidepressant use in pregnant women (Rapaport 2015). The risk appears to be small early in pregnancy, but climbs in the second and third trimesters, when expectant mothers who take antidepressants are nearly 90 percent more likely to deliver a newborn with ASD than those who avoid them. Selective serotonin reuptake inhibitors (SSRI), mentioned in earlier chapters and available in widely prescribed Paxil, Prozac, Zoloft, and Celexa, appear to carry the greatest risk. Mildly depressed pregnant women may be able to improve their condition with exercise, but serious cases require medical intervention. Even were an expectant mother able to prevent ASD in her newborn by eschewing antidepressants, this action makes little sense when avoidance compounds depression.

Over the counter (OTC) medicines may not be benign given that the Danish National Birth Cohort, an ongoing study of pregnancy complications and newborn diseases and disorders, asserts that expectant mothers who use acetaminophen, a pain reducer and Tylenol's active ingredient, even once during pregnancy have a 50 percent greater chance of having a baby with ASD than those who do not take it. The risk increases with each additional tablet but only in cases where newborns with ASD grow more hyperactive and impulsive as they mature. Other ASD cases appear to be unrelated to acetaminophen consumption during pregnancy. These findings may prompt women never to take acetaminophen while pregnant in hopes of preventing ASD in babies, but these hopes may be unrealistic.

ASD PREVENTION STRATEGIES DURING DELIVERY OF NEWBORNS

Medically induced labor may cause or contribute to ASD in newborns, especially boys (Gregory 2013). Among chemicals used in induction is naturally occurring oxytocin, whose benefits are noted in earlier chapters and which should not be withheld when pregnant women need help stimulating contractions. Of the more than 625,000 babies born in North Carolina from 1990 to 1998, the boys were 35 percent more likely to have ASD when their mothers used oxytocin and other labor inducing chemicals than the boys born without these interventions. These data suggest that women who avoid taking labor inducing chemicals during delivery may prevent ASD in newborn boys in some instances, but this strategy does not work in all cases. That is, abstinence from oxytocin or another labor inducing chemical does not prevent ASD in all newborns.

Some births are cesarean in reference to the surgical technique cesarean section or C-section, a procedure to save mother and baby when the baby does not pass easily through the birth canal. Women who have a C-section are more likely to deliver a baby with ASD than women who do not (Curran 2015). The article does not state that C-sections cause ASD. Rather a faulty gene or genes may cause both ASD in newborns and the need for a C-section in their mothers during delivery. In this scenario, women who do not have a C-section do not prevent ASD in newborns because the baby was not at risk of having ASD from the harmful gene or genes.

CONCLUSION

The rules of evidence in the sciences and medicine dictate that empirical evidence alone can prove whether ASD can be prevented. Preventative guidelines, numerous but not ironclad, center on the expectant mother. She may modify the diet, avoid toxins, and strengthen healthy habits to include exercise, the breathing of clean air, and repudiation of electronic devices. Avoiding nicotine confers many benefits and should be pursued whether or not its absence prevents ASD. An expectant mother might err on the side of caution by minimizing the use of OTC medicines like acetaminophen. Where antibiotics and antidepressants are necessary, a pregnant woman should not eschew them in hopes of preventing ASD in her baby. She might favor a natural birth because it might prevent ASD in some newborns. Whatever a natural birth's value, a C-section is sometimes necessary. The next chapter turns from prevention—an issue full of debates, arguments, counterarguments, interpretations of evidence, possibilities for persuasion or profits, opportunities for basic and applied research, and attempts to influence science and medicine—to other issues and controversies that shape knowledge about and attitudes toward ASD.

REFERENCES

Ansel, Karen. 2018. "Autism Spectrum Disorders (ASD) and Diet." *Academy of Nutrition and Dietetics.* April 2. https://www.eatright.org/health/diseases-and -conditions/autism/nutrition-for-your-child-with-autism-spectrum -disorder-asd.

Benson, Dana. 2016. "Study to Investigate Connection Between Antibiotic Use and Autism Symptoms." Baylor College of Medicine. December 1. https://www.bcm.edu/news/pathology-and-immunology/study -connection-between-antibiotics-austism.

Buffington, S. A., G. V. Di Prisco, T. A. Auchtung, N. J. Ajami, J. F. Petrosino, and M. Costa-Mattioli. 2016. "Microbial Reconstitution Reverses Maternal Diet-Induced Social and Synaptic Deficits in Offspring." *Cell* 165, no. 7 (June): 1762–1775.

Curran, E. A., C. Dalman, P. M. Kearney, L. C. Kenny, J. F. Cryan, T. G. Dinan, and A. S. Khashan. 2015. "Association between Obstetric Mode of Delivery and Autism Spectrum Disorder: A Population-Based Sibling Design Study." *Journal of the American Medical Associate Psychiatry* 72, no. 9 (September): 935–942.

Dunckley, Victoria L. 2016. "Autism and Screen Time: Special Brains, Special Risks." *Psychology Today.* December 31. https://www .psychologytoday.com/us/blog/mental-wealth/201612/autism-and -screen-time-special-brains-special-risks.

Eliasen, M., J. S. Tolstrup, A. M. Nybo Andersen, M. Gronbaek, J. Olsen, and K. Strandberg-Laresen. 2010. "Prenatal Alcohol Exposure and Autistic Spectrum Disorders—APopulation-Based Prospective Study of 80,552 Children and Their Mothers." *International Journal of Epidemiology* 39, no. 4 (August): 1074–1081.

Fallon, J. 2005. "Could One of the Most Widely Prescribed Antibiotics Amoxicillin/Clavulanate 'Augmentin' Be a Risk Factor for Autism?" *Medical Hypotheses* 64, no. 2: 312–315.

Gregory, S. G., R. Anthopolos, C. E. Osgood, C. A. Grotegut, and M. L. Miranda. 2013. "Association of Autism with Induced or Augmented Childbirth in North Carolina Birth Record (1990–1998) and Education Research (1997–2007) Databases." *Journal of the American Medical Association Pediatrics* 167, no. 10 (October): 959–966.

IQAir. n.d. "Air Pollution and Autism." https://www.iqair.com/newsroom/air-pollution-and-autism.

Jung, Yonwoo, Angela M. Lee, Sherry A. McKee, and Marina R. Picciotto. 2017. "Maternal Smoking and Autism Spectrum Disorder: Meta-Analysis with Population Smoking Metrics as Moderators." *Scientific Reports* 7:4315.

McDonnell, Maureen H. 2010. "What Can Be Done to Prevent Autism Now?" Pathways to Family Wellness. http://pathwaystofamilywellness.org/Informed-Choice/what-can-be-done-to-prevent-autism-now.html.

Moninger, Jeannette. n.d. "Pregnancy and Autism: What You Need to Know." *Parents.* https://www.parents.com/pregnancy/my-baby/pregnancy-and-autism-what-you-need-to-know/.

National Institutes of Health. 2005. "Autism and Genes." Bethesda, MD: National Institute of Health. NIH Pub, no. 05–5590. https://files.eric.ed.gov/fulltext/ED485722.pdf.

National Institutes of Health. 2008. "Autism Risk Higher in People with Gene Variant." January. https://www.nih.gov/news-events/news-releases/autism-risk-higher-people-gene-variant.

Oken, Emily, and David C. Bellinger. 2008. "Fish Consumption, Methylmercury and Child Neurodevelopment." *Current Opinion in Pediatrics* 20, no. 2 (April): 178–183.

Rapaport, Lisa. 2015. "Antidepressants in Pregnancy Tied to Autism." *Reuters Health.* December 14. https://www.reuters.com/article/us-health-autism-antidepressants/antidepressants-in-pregnancy-tied-to-autism-idUSKBN0TX22C20151214.

Shelton, Janie F., Estella M. Geraghty, Daniel J. Tancredi, Lora D. Delwiche, Rebecca J. Schmidt, Beate Ritz, Robin L. Hansen, and Irva Hertz-Picciotto. 2014. "Neurodevelopmental Disorders and Prenatal Residential Proximity to Agricultural Pesticides: The CHARGE Study." *Environmental Health Perspectives* 122:1103–1109.

Sifferlin, Alexandra. 2016. "The Link between Mosquito Spraying and Autism." *Time,* April 30. http://time.com/4313156/mosquito-spraying-autism-pesticides/.

Singer, A. B., A. S. Aylsworth, C. Cordero, L. A. Croen, C. DiGuiseppi, M. D. Fallin, A. H. Herring, et al. 2017. "Prenatal Alcohol Exposure in Relation to Autism Spectrum Disorder: Findings from the Study to Explore Early Development (SEED)." *Pediatric and Perinatal Epidemiology* 31, no. 6 (November): 573–582.

Tweed, Lindsey, Nancy Connolly, and Amy Beaulieu. 2009. "Interventions for Autism Spectrum Disorders: State of Evidence." Augusta: Muskie School of Public Service and the Maine Department of Health and Human Services. http://digitalcommons.usm.maine.edu/cyf/7/.

Velasquez-Manoff, Moises. 2012. "An Immune Disorder at the Root of Autism." *New York Times*, August 25. https://www.nytimes.com/2012/08/26/opinion/sunday/immune-disorders-and-autism.html.

Vinkhuyzen, A. A. E., Darryl W. Eyles, Thomas H. J. Burne, Laura M. E. Blanken, Claudia J. Kruithof, Frank Verhulst, Tonya White, et al. 2017. "Gestational Vitamin D Deficiency and Autism Spectrum Disorder." *British Journal of Psychiatry* 3, no. 2 (March): 85–90.

Volknow, N. D., G. J. Wang, S. H. Kollins, T. L. Wigal, J. H. Newcorn, F. Telang, J. S. Fowler, et al. 2009. "Evaluating Dopamine Reward Pathway in ADHD: Clinical Implications." *Journal of the American Medical Association* 302, no. 10 (September), 1084–1091.

Yau, V. M., P. G. Green, C. P. Alaimo, C. K. Yoshida, M. Lutsky, G. C. Windham, G. Delorenze, et al. 2014. "Prenatal and Neonatal Peripheral Blood Mercury Levels and Autism Spectrum Disorders." *Environmental Research* 133 (August): 294–303.

9

Issues and Controversies

Like anything complex and worth effort, exploration, and thought, autism spectrum disorder (ASD) has plenty of controversies and salient issues. The chief controversy has centered on whether vaccines cause ASD. This tumult, peaking in the early 2000s, is less noisy now because the scientific and medical communities have rebuffed speculation. Nonetheless sounds continue to reverberate in some quarters for various reasons including a Bible literalist backlash that tries to pit God's authority against the human frailties evident in all undertakings including science and medicine. The vaccine under fire was an old but effective version of a measles, mumps, and rubella (MMR) vaccine, which continues to attract attention. A controversy that remains heated concerns the use of applied behavioral analysis therapy (ABA) on children with ASD with ASD. In addition to these controversies, problems are evident in the divisive issues that put ASD in the larger contexts of the economy, education, race, geography, and public attitudes and prejudices. All facets of these issues cannot receive treatment here.

CONTROVERSIES

Vaccination

The advent of vaccinations marked a watershed in history by setting previously unattainable standards of safety and effectiveness against infectious diseases. The initial triumph against the viral disease smallpox fueled additional discoveries that led to an array of vaccines against several pathogenic bacteria and viruses and, in the process, changed almost everything about human existence. Vaccination is so important that many countries, including the United States, compel it to prevent the appalling child mortality that long plagued humans.

Despite the importance of vaccination, opponents worldwide can exempt themselves or their children from the requirement. These exemptions can be confusing because they vary by country and, in the United States, by state. In the United States, states may grant exemptions on religious, personal, or medical grounds. States are most reluctant to grant medical exemptions, though no citizen may presume automatic exemption in the other two cases. Variations in vaccination laws and exemptions defy encapsulation (Walkinshaw 2011). This context, leading to confusion and suspicion, has engendered controversy in the United States and elsewhere.

A single event precipitated a near-revolt against vaccination on the suspicion that it might cause ASD in children, hostility that has yet to vanish. A study published in *The Lancet* (Wakefield et al. 1998) targeted the MMR vaccine, whose safety had been questioned as early as the 1980s because critics questioned the process of adding mercury as preservation for storage. Mercury works as a preservative because, being toxic, it delays the growth of any pathogen in the vaccine. Additionally, mercury is the only metal to be a liquid at room temperature and so is readily mixed with any other preservatives. These advantages are real, but cannot hinder critics from pinpointing mercury's obvious toxicity, a fact known for centuries. That is, the critics were correct, but their objections failed to override the fact that this MMR vaccine worked. By 2001, mercury had been replaced by other preservatives in almost all vaccines.

Wakefield's paper focused on the parents and physicians of eight developmentally disabled children in a sample of twelve. The parents pointed to the MMR vaccine as initiator of their children's misbehaviors. Wakefield and coauthors described several signs and symptoms that led them to coin a new disorder, autistic enterocolitis, which they conjectured to be an inflammation of the digestive tract. Upon the paper's publication, Wakefield convened a press conference at the hospital that employed him.

The conflagration was not immediate, but once it began to smolder Wakefield intensified the flames. American model and actress Jenny McCarthy took up arms in the belief that her two-and-a-half-year-old son had contracted ASD from a series of vaccinations. Her narrative of her son's ordeal and his doctors' indifference and incompetence united with her celebrity to galvanize both media and public. Her fad treatments for her son, three books, and agitation among parents followed. Other popular

American actors, including Robert De Niro and Jim Carrey, joined the movement, though their exertions were inconspicuous at the time. Only since the controversy's debacle have their voices lingered long enough to be heard. Whatever their impact, these efforts piggybacked on McCarthy's to amplify a hysteria that led many Americans to believe that doctors were forcing unsafe vaccines upon them and their children as part of a malevolent conspiracy. Parents in the United States, United Kingdom, Italy, Japan, and Australia flouted vaccination laws in the belief that they were protecting their children from ASD. Such vitriol led some unvaccinated children to die from diseases that these vaccines would have prevented.

Worse traumas might have ensued but for the intervention of British journalist Brian Deer, who in 2004 exposed Wakefield as a con man and his study as fraudulent. Deer demonstrated that before publication of the notorious paper, Wakefield had sought a patent for a new MMR vaccine and so stood to gain financially by discrediting the old one. Moreover, a law firm had paid him to undertake the study and had sent its clients to him for confirmation that the old MMR vaccine had caused their children's ASD. Armed with this verdict, the firm filed several suits against the vaccine's maker. In addition, Wakefield falsified data from his study of the 12 children and had never received approval to conduct it in the first place, despite his use of invasive procedures against disabled children who could not advocate for themselves. Wakefield shared none of this information with *Lancet* editors. Several of the paper's coauthors confessed in 2004 that no evidence implicated the old MMR vaccine as a cause of ASD. In 2010, *The Lancet*'s editors retracted the paper, a rare action given that retraction forever taints a journal. Afterwards, other studies documented the MMR vaccine's safety, further debunking the claim that it caused ASD.

Applied Behavioral Analysis (ABA) Therapy

Earlier chapters articulated the belief among some mental health specialists that ABA is the best non-pharmacological therapy available to children with ASD. Yet counter narratives are emerging from parents who express fear and alarm at what their children with ASD endure during therapy and from adults with ASD who say they suffered cruelties while undergoing it as children. Such criticisms come when ABA is the most widespread therapy for treating ASD (Raeburn-Devita 2016).

In this context, note the degree to which ABA has penetrated all levels of educational psychology and therapies for people with ASD with ASD from preschoolers to adults. ABA has been recommended as early as possible in childhood and in long durations to achieve the best outcomes (Granpeesheh et al. 2009). Such recommendations have enabled ABA to infiltrate schools, corroborating the judgment that it is the stellar non-pharmacological treatment.

Critics charge that ABA attempts to make people with ASD "normal." That is, ABA seeks to compel people with ASD to behave within the narrow limits of what conforms to societal expectations. Many adults with ASD who suffered under ABA's tyranny as children instead want therapists and the public to accept them as they are, rather than disdain them as abnormal. They are different, not aberrant or deviant. No therapy, including ABA, should force people with ASD or anyone else to mimic robots. Other critics brand ABA a type of aggressive marketing that leads parents to fear that their ASD child will never improve without it. This tactic stokes guilt and distress so that inaction is tantamount to admitting culpability and poor parenting. This heavy hand tightens wherever government mandates restrict options. Note that Medicare and Medicaid, as administered by most states, cover ABA but reimburse the cost of other therapies only partly if at all. For instance, California requires that Medicare and Medicaid recipients pay all non-ABA therapy costs.

Despite these concerns, ABA has had decades to build momentum and support. Founder Norwegian American psychologist and University of California, Los Angeles (UCLA) professor Ole Ivar Lovaas crusaded during the 1960s against warehousing people with ASD in institutions for life. The result was a noble ambition concretized in ABA, which he invented to give people with ASD an opportunity to live and work outside institutions. The most successful lived on their own in an apartment or home. In his first attempts, Lovaas boasted that ABA decreased harmful behaviors and increased sociability and language. These gains boosted intelligence quotients (IQ). Even children with marked cognitive impairments succeeded in school beyond parents and teachers' expectations. Those in first grade sometimes merited promotion to second grade.

But early successes stalled whenever ABA therapists, following protocol, yelled at, slapped, or even jolted ASD children with electricity. In other cases, therapists treated them like animals by dangling food before them. The reward could only be gotten by following ABA directives. As critics began to oppose it on these grounds, the goal of preparing people with ASD for independence and work retreated as people doubted that ABA could impart any useful skills. For example, children with ASD could learn through intensive drills to make eye contact with a therapist or ask his or her name. But these skills did not extend beyond therapy because these children seldom made eye contact with strangers, peers, or even acquaintances; when requesting a name, they failed to await a response, indicating no understanding of what they were asking.

In fundamental ways, ABA was neither science nor medicine because until 2010 no researcher had published a paper with data from a randomized trial. In effect, ABA advocates expected parent, child, and public to abandon their critical faculties and accept that it must work because they said so. That year, the U.S. Department of Education, examining 58 studies, rated only one as having an adequate research design. It measured only meager improvements in children who underwent ABA.

ISSUES

The Economy

ASD's important issues revolve around troubling disparities. Economic trends favor neurotypical job seekers and employees over ASD counterparts, and as the chasm between the two widens, it becomes too easy to blame people with ASD for lagging behind neurotypical workers, managers, and investors. Abrasive commentators claim that people with ASD and the disabled in general must be deficient to fare so poorly in the competition for jobs, wealth, and other resources. These matters demonstrate that connections between ASD and the economy are full of debate and divergent perspectives so that the two are controversial as well as crucial.

Other economic factors hinge on employability and are well known. Job seekers with ASD are less likely than neurotypical people to excel at interviews. The human resources director may be unable to pinpoint why she does not favor ASD candidates beyond acknowledging that they discomfort her. People with ASD may sense this discomfort and try to adapt by masking their signs and symptoms and not divulging their diagnosis. Once hired, assuming they have convinced the human resources director of their worth or hidden their shortcomings, employees with ASD may not hold a job long when coworkers find them creepy because they frown or display no emotion at jokes and smile at the narration of sad stories. Consequently, many people with ASD move from job to job (Imam 2013).

Economic matters can be separated neither from turmoil in public education that leads to bullying and intense shame nor from family problems, substandard living accommodations, public prejudices, dismal self-esteem, ASD comorbidities, inadequate government efforts to treat ASD and other disabilities, and an absence of mentors and role models especially for adults. All these issues cannot receive treatment in this chapter; instead the analysis clings to just the economy, if such attempts are possible, even as it acknowledges that people with ASD have many problems. These economic, educational, generational, psychological, and health problems snowball so that people with ASD and other disabled people feel no self worth because too many others denigrate them as "moochers" and "welfare leeches." Because of poverty, many disabled people cannot afford decent housing and must trudge through a swamp of noxious rentals.

Other issues stemming from the connections between economic matters and ASD cannot be untangled here.

The poor are more likely than the rich to have attention deficit hyperactivity disorder (ADHD) and asthma, but less likely to have ASD (Pulcini et al. 2017; Durkin et al. 2017). These findings might be an artifact of economic and medical circumstances; the poor are unlikely to consult a doctor because of inability to pay and so are seldom diagnosed with ASD, whereas the opposite dynamic applies to the rich. Other studies support this inverse correlation but do not resolve the problem of the poor's infrequent doctor visits. Although the link between ASD and poverty can be interpreted as meaningful or accidental, one study concluded that cognitively impaired children are diagnosed with ASD just as often as children with average intelligence irrespective of parents' income (Durkin et al. 2017). Here again, it is difficult to extract the proper conclusion from these data because most ASD cases are diagnosed by or before age two. But most children this young are not in school and so cannot have been observed by teachers, counselors, administrators, nurses, and other personnel. Instead the onus of recognizing the red flags and going to the doctor falls on parents, and the consensus holds that poor parents seek medical care for their children less often than do affluent parents. This reality reverts to the aforementioned probability that the poor are less often diagnosed with ASD than the rich. These complications are germane to countries (like the United States) with private sector health care; in countries like Sweden, France, Canada, and a handful of others with national health care, where everyone should have equal access to medical care, no evidence links ASD to either poverty or wealth. Causation cannot be proved either way.

Among developed countries, contradiction emerges when the emphasis is on Hong Kong and Singapore, the pair ranking first and second worldwide in percentage of urbanites. Hong Kong has the world's highest proportion of people with ASD (Charron 2017). Logic dictates that ASD's geography must be more urban than rural. Yet Singapore, having less than one-fifth Hong Kong's percentage of ASD urbanites, seems to demonstrate that ASD must afflict more people in the countryside than in the city. Nonetheless, several highly urbanized nations, including South Korea, the United States, and Japan, have the second, third, and fourth highest percentages of people with ASD, reverting to what might be called the Hong Kong syndrome in which ASD may be more urban than rural. Another explanation for urbanism may be that these nations, all affluent, are better able to attend to medical needs, providing opportunities to diagnose ASD. Yet this explanation does not square with the U.S. healthcare system.

This phenomenon aligns with research that pinpoints ASD in the south and west portions of the United States, with Alabama having the country's largest percentage of eight-year-olds with ASD and Colorado the third largest (Baio 2014). By many measures, Alabama is a poor state and thus unlikely to see many patients. The state therefore should not over diagnose ASD, meaning that Alabama's ASD percentages should tilt toward understatement, not exaggeration. Because Alabama is rural, ASD appears to concentrate in America's countryside. People with ASD, especially children, also concentrate in rural Appalachia, where thousands wait years for treatment and those on Medicaid cannot get treatment in West Virginia because so many practitioners do not accept Medicaid (Lofton 2016). These factors reinforce the conclusions that ASD concentrates in the countryside and among the poor.

Longevity

Longevity's importance cannot be understated because biology and medicine measure success or failure partly by tabulating lifespans for different ethnicities, races, genders, people of various genetic endowments, ancestries, upbringings, sexual orientations, activity levels, exposures to toxins, hygienic habits, geographies, religions, belief systems, tendencies toward or away from gregariousness, social skills, and dietary preferences. These measurements extend to groups divided by income, occupation, investment prowess, work history, putative work ethic, education, or some combination of all six. In short, longevity preoccupies the sciences and medicine.

Scrutiny extends to people with ASD, who on average appear to live 20 fewer years than neurotypical people. In some cases their lives are even briefer (Underwood 2016). Cognitively impaired people with ASD perish three decades earlier than people free from ASD and mental impairment. These disparities are chilling because adults with ASD (men and women), even those without any cognitive impairment, kill themselves nine times more frequently than neurotypical people, a rate that climbs even higher when men are excluded from the tabulation, meaning that women with ASD are more prone than any other group, healthy or disabled in some way, to commit suicide. In addition, people with ASD are roughly 2.5 times more likely to die early from a terminal disease than the average neurotypical person because they have trouble articulating their worries to doctors, who assume that nothing is wrong until death is too near to avert (Hirvikoski et al. 2016). Accidents claim other lives when children and adults with ASD wander away from supervision only to drown in a pool or other body of water (Underwood 2016). Another staggering calculation estimates that mentally impaired people with ASD are nearly 40 times more likely than neurotypicals to die of epilepsy or a related condition (Cusak et al. 2016). The report documents that people with ASD die earlier than neurotypicals from a lengthy list of diseases and conditions, possibly because late diagnoses are too prevalent (Underwood 2016). The most sinister finding may be that the average adult with ASD dies at age 54 (Mills 2016), though some claim that early ASD mortality is an artifact of accidents like drowning that artificially diminish longevity (National Autism Association n.d.). Yet if twice the percentage of people with ASD than the average neurotypical person dies early, then their lifespan must shorten. Death is not artificial.

Race

Race informs and sharpens ASD's disparities; medical practitioners have ignored blacks and other minorities with ASD (Silberman 2016). This problem began early, when Austrian American physician and ASD pioneer Leo Kanner failed to study a single African American with ASD in his landmark 1943 paper referenced in earlier chapters. Of the eleven subjects, nine were "Anglo-Saxon" and the remaining two were Jewish. All came from affluent families, whose parents Kanner labeled scientists, academics, attorneys, and physicians, all of whom were thought to occupy the apex of success and educational attainment. This adulation of white professionals infected scholarship for decades. For example, twentieth century psychologist, professor, and researcher Victor Sanua supposed that ASD was the price to pay for Western civilization's advances, particularly technology. In other words, professionals and technocrats had succeeded too well, bringing ASD upon them. This may partly explain why some doctors fretted over vaccines, and why so many Americans feared that these pathogen protectors might cause ASD. If ASD afflicts white professionals, the source of technological progress, then their opposites (minorities, especially blacks) must be too retrograde to have it.

This logic dictates that if minorities cannot have ASD, then another malady or maladies must mimic its signs and symptoms. Accordingly, doctors posited that conditions like minimal cognition, ADHD, or a behavioral problem afflicted minorities, especially children. Minority parents decried these faulty premises and the neglect of blacks, Latinos, and East Asians with undiagnosed or late diagnosed ASD, but prejudices linger. In a genetic context, some scientists and medical researchers believe that minorities might have a gene or genes that shield them from ASD. Impervious to it, minorities need no medical intervention even when they display ASD signs and symptoms. This perverse logic is evident in the reality that minority children receive an ASD diagnosis when they are roughly two years older than their white counterparts at the time of diagnosis. The consensus, reiterated throughout ASD literature, holds that diagnosis and treatment delays irreparably harm children with ASD.

CONCLUSION

Controversies mar the study of ASD; diagnosis; treatment; management; outcomes; economic, social, and racial dynamics; and public sentiments, attitudes, and perceptions. In the case of minorities, too often ASD signs and symptoms are dismissed as some other affliction. Stereotypes frequently silence legitimate concerns about ASD from minority parents, their children, other relatives, friends, coworkers, and acquaintances. Thoughts that technological advances have led white elites to develop ASD may implicate vaccines, an essential product of science, medicine, and technology. These memes may have undergirded the controversy over whether vaccines cause ASD, a topic examined earlier. Vaccines are not the lone controversy. ABA is in some camps the most effective talk therapy, but others deem it insensitive and cruel. These controversies and issues play out against the backdrop of the global economy, which influences many facets of ASD including health, educational, and geographic disparities, with education a recurrent subject. The final chapter does not dim the focus on crucial issues, including the current state of research and predictions about the direction of science and medicine and possible changes in attitudes and laws about people with ASD as the twenty-first century continues to unfold.

REFERENCES

Baio, Jon. 2014. "Prevalence of Autism Spectrum Disorder among Children Aged 8 Years—Autism and Developmental Disabilities Monitoring Network, 11 Sites, United States, 2010." *Surveillance Summaries* 63, SS02 (March 28): 1–21.

Charron, Robyn. 2017. "Autism Rates across the Developed World." *Focus for Health,* August 28. https://www.focusforhealth.org/autism-rates -across-the-developed-world/.

Cusak, James, Simon Shaw, Jon Spiers, and Rebecca Sterry. 2016. "Personal Tragedies, Public Crisis." Autistica. www.autismeurope.org/wp -content/uploads/2017/08/personal-tragedies-public-crisis.pdf.

Durkin, Maureen S., Matthew J. Maenner, Jon Baio, D. Christensen, J. Daniels, R. Fitzgerald, P. Imm, et al. 2017. "Autism Spectrum Disorder among US Children (2002-2010): Socioeconomic, Racial, and Ethnic Disparities." *American Journal of Public Health* 107, no. 11 (November), 1818–1826.

Granpeesheh, Doreen, Dennis R. Dixon, Jonathan Tarbox, Andrew M. Kaplan, and Arthur E. Wilke. 2009. "The Effects of Age and Treatment Intensity on Behavioral Intervention for Children with

Autism Spectrum Disorders." *Research in Autism Spectrum Disorders*, 3, no. 4 (October –December): 1014–1022.

Hirvikoski T., E. Mittendorfer-Rutz, M. Boman, H. Larsson, P. Lichtenstein, and S. Bölte. 2016. "Premature Mortality in Autism Spectrum Disorder." *British Journal of Psychiatry* 208, no. 3: 232–238.

Imam, Jareen. 2013. "The Reality of Finding a Job with Autism." *CNN*, May 6. https://www.cnn.com/2013/04/30/health/irpt-autism-in-the-workplace/index.html.

Lofton, Kara Leigh. 2016. "Autism Services Lacking for West Virginia Families." *West Virginia Public Broadcasting*, April 6. http://wvpublic.org/post/autism-services-lacking-west-virginia-families.

Mills, David. 2016. "Why People with Autism Die at a Much Younger Age." Healthline, March 25. https://www.healthline.com/health-news/why-people-with-autism-die-at-younger-age.

National Autism Association. n.d. "Autism Fact Sheet." http://nationalautismassociation.org/resources/autism-fact-sheet/.

Pulcini, Christian D., Bonnie T. Zima, Kelly J. Kelleher, and Amy J. Houtrow. 2017. "Poverty and Trends in 3 Common Chronic Disorders." *Pediatrics* 139, no. 3 (March): e20162539.

Raeburn-Devita, Elizabeth. 2016. "Is the Most Common Therapy for Autism Cruel?" *The Atlantic*, August 11. https://www.theatlantic.com/health/archive/2016/08/aba-autism-controversy/495272/.

Silberman, Steve. 2016. "The Invisibility of Black Autism." *Undark*, May 17. https://undark.org/article/invisibility-black-autism/.

Underwood, Emily. 2016. "People on Autism Spectrum Die 18 Years Younger Than Average." *Science*, March 17. http://www.sciencemag.org/news/2016/03/people-autism-spectrum-die-18-years-younger-average.

Wakefield, A. J., S. H. Murch, A. Anthony, J. Linnell, D. M. Casson, M. Malik, M. Berelowitz, et al. 1998. "Ileal-Lymphoid-Nodular Hyperplasia, Non-Specific Colitis, and Pervasive Developmental Disorder in Children." *The Lancet* 351, no. 9103 (February): 637–641.

Walkinshaw, Erin. 2011. "Mandatory Vaccinations: The International Landscape." *Canadian Medical Association Journal* 183, no. 16 (November): e1167–e1168.

10

Current Research and Future Directions

As climbers near the summit, they want to be sure of the terrain underfoot and their distance from the peak. This inquiry likewise ends by surveying the current state of research and attempting to predict the future landscape of autism spectrum disorder (ASD), which will surely point toward several paths, all of which cannot be trod. One trail may lead to more intensive and expensive research, though restrictions on federal spending may truncate this route. These contributions are just what researchers will need to fuel the next generation of medicines and other therapies. Another trail will probably explore societal issues including public attitudes and legal advancements to protect and better the lives of people with ASD and their caretakers. As does current legislation, these laws will surely shape public education and parental rights. Under these circumstances, future laws will continue to affect children with ASD in public schools, while those in private schools may benefit from attempts to replicate or surpass public education in accommodating new directives. The additional burden of record keeping and resentment toward federal laws that mandate changes without funding their implementation (unfunded mandates) will continue to frustrate school administrators and their employees, who already feel themselves pulled in too many directions. Whatever the effects on children, new and expanded laws will not likely ignore the adult with ASD as researchers and the public grow increasingly aware that he or she deserves more vigorous study, attention, and protections. Expanding their

reach, new laws will almost certainly affect hiring and employment practices, which adults with ASD believe to be antiquated and biased against
them. In this regard the Americans with Disabilities Act (ADA) may gain
additional powers targeted, perhaps aggressively, at employers, though
businesses may push back. Such behavior will exacerbate longstanding differences in economic policies between Republicans and Democrats. As
battle lines are drawn, differences will smolder locally and nationwide,
igniting fires wherever disagreements are sharpest.

CURRENT RESEARCH

The Gene

Earlier chapters emphasized that genes dictate much about ASD's onset
and severity, even granting the environment a role in modifying the severity. Biological determinism, if such language is permissible, has required
and continues to require intensive genetic research if scientists and medical experts are ever to understand ASD in enough detail to permit derivation of new and enhanced therapies to minimize each ASD person's
limitations and maximize his or her strengths. In other words, current and
future research may inaugurate an era when doctors can tailor therapies of
all types to the needs of each child, adolescent, and adult with ASD.

Current research concentrates in two areas, the first being genomics. In
conception and application, genomic research requires scientists to display
many strengths, including an ability to define the structure and function
of a genome and to posit how it came to be, the second task being the
domain of evolutionary genetics. These strands of genomic knowledge
should allow scientists to map and alter a genome with far reaching effects.
Such alteration is now possible only to a limited extent in humans and is
the purview of gene therapy (mentioned in earlier chapters), a branch of
which is genetic engineering, whose potential to modify species should be
enormous given its usefulness in agriculture alone. But because many people fear genetic engineering or at least its possible consequences, it is
unlikely to apply directly to humans. Were we to use genetic engineering
to modify ourselves in the future, many aspects of what we call reality
would change, revolutionizing what we are and believe and how we act.
Even without these sweeping changes, uncontroversial versions of gene
therapy, when sufficiently advanced, should allow physicians to cure ASD.
The cure will not likely occur in the near term but may nonetheless mark a
watershed in history when it arrives. In other words, and contrary to the
advice never to put all eggs in one basket, gene therapy is the nest that
should hold the vast preponderance of eggs.

Just as an international team of scientists launched and completed what might be termed the first stage of the Human Genome Project (HGP) by mapping the sequence of nucleotide bases in every human gene, the Autism Genome Project (AGP), arguably the most ambitious undertaking in ASD science and medicine, seeks to identify every gene that causes or contributes to ASD's onset and severity. Such a goal surpasses what the HGP has achieved so far. The project's complexity can only be glimpsed here by indicating that many genes shape the expression of one or a group of genes, that not all genes code for proteins because many are chemically inactive, that many genes are imperfect because they have mutations and because these mutations almost always harm an organism, that biotechnology (genetic engineering) allows scientists to transfer a gene or genes from one organism to another, that the results of such transfers cannot always be predicted, and that cloning allows a genome to be replicated in an offspring with unpredictable results. All these factors but cloning have received attention in earlier chapters. Other possibilities exist so that the task of identifying every harmful (mutant or mutated) ASD gene involves many contingencies because scientists do not yet know how biotechnology and other genetic manipulations might shape the function of such genes. At least hypothetically, genetic alterations should be able to restore harmful genes to a benign or even a beneficial state. Such advances should put science and medicine on the threshold of a cure.

The foregoing sharpens the focus on harmful genes. Not only must scientists identify them all as the AGP progresses, but they must also learn how these harmful genes work in every detail to enable their suppression. Better would be the transformation of these genes from harmful to beneficial. The lone scientist or physician cannot achieve this ambition. Accordingly, the AGP is what historians of science, medicine, and technology call "big science," assembling worldwide the genomes of some 2,000 families with at least two children with ASD (Autism Speaks 2011). When complete, this assemblage might be the world's largest repository of genomes involved in ASD's onset and severity. The project has already pinpointed several faulty genes with additional discoveries expected in coming years. If successful, it should accelerate gene therapy, the aforementioned tool for curing ASD. Because ASD varies, sometimes dramatically, in onset and severity, the tool likely must construct many cures, each specific to each person with ASD.

The Brain

At the core a neurological condition, ASD has required and continues to demand probing into the machinery of the brain and other parts of the central nervous system (CNS), another example of the degree to which ASD's biology shapes research. Studies pursue various neurological aspects including defects in the brain's pruning of synapses between neurons. Earlier chapters mentioned the phenomenon given that the brain develops in complex ways, in which two stages may be identified. First, as the fetus takes shape in the womb, the brain enlarges to produce more neurons and more synapses between them. This process continues after birth, when the brain grows quickly in its initial years. Once this process has peaked, the brain consolidates these gains and in fact reduces the number of synapses, apparently in the drive toward greater efficiency.

But the ASD brain is different because pruning slows down when it should hold steady, resulting in too many synapses for efficiency. These extra synapses contribute to ASD's onset and severity, requiring research into why pruning slows too much too soon. Borrowing an earlier theme, genetic research is necessary to clarify why pruning goes awry, usually during adolescence, retarding learning and socialization. Returning to yet another earlier theme, this faulty pruning occurs in both ASD and schizophrenia, conditions that have long confused researchers and clinicians because of similar signs and symptoms. In other words, clarification of pruning's genetics should illuminate the development and potentially the treatment of both maladies. Research that can achieve this twin aim is valuable and so constitutes an important line of research, now and in the future.

For example, the drug rapamycin has the potential to stop mice brains from displaying ASD-like attributes because they no longer slow the reduction of synapses (Belluck 2014). If the drug works in humans, it may inaugurate a new era in ASD treatment, though rapamycin has potentially life-threatening side effects. Moreover, mice do not go through adolescence in the way that humans do. In fact, the maturation that occurs during human adolescence seems vaster and more sweeping, at least cognitively, than what occurs in other animals. In addition, a brain receptor may begin adolescent pruning, a finding that motivates current research into the mechanism that actuates and regulates this receptor (Scripps Research Institute 2016). Given the foregoing, this receptor must be able to prevent pruning from slowing too soon to be worth scientific and medical scrutiny. Science and medicine, in seeking to know why the receptor functions as it does at the tempo that it does, move ahead with this agenda. At stake are the education and treatment of adolescents with ASD and possibly schizophrenia, another potential boon making this research crucial now and into the future. The mystery deepens given that ASD arises very early in childhood and might be present in the simplest, most basic form at conception because ASD's faulty genes must activate in some fashion in the zygote; on the other hand schizophrenia seldom manifests before age sixteen, leading to the conundrum that if the same genes are responsible for both ASD and schizophrenia, they nonetheless switch on at different times in each, as though one movement of a single switch could turn on a lightbulb at dawn and again at noon. That single flick of a switch must be able to pulse electricity into the lightbulb at dawn and again at noon. Putting aside the electricity analogy, this mechanism is not understood in medicine and so should heighten ASD genetic research's importance today and tomorrow.

ASD's genetic roots continue to shape the emerging tree of research. Mutant versions of PTEN (phosphatase and tensin homolog) are implicated in causing or contributing to some ASD signs and symptoms (Scripps Research Institute 2015). The mutations stimulate the production of too many neurons and glia in the cortex so that overall the brain grows too large, a phenomenon mentioned earlier. As do numerous studies in ASD and other afflictions, this study focused on mice in hopes that the findings might apply to ASD in humans. Research discovered that apoptosis (cell death) sometimes proceeds too fast in mice brains; even though such rapidity should harm mice, it seems to stop the brain from making too many neurons and synapses, halting ASD before it harms cognition. In other words, a paradox results in which a dangerous excess (acceleration of apoptosis) creates a healthful outcome (normal cognition). More studies are necessary to clarify why what ought to endanger health improves it in mice that should display the rodent version of ASD.

Whatever the full effects, they highlight the centrality of ASD genetics related to brain development. The brain can become neither too large (macrocephaly) nor too small (microcephaly). Some children with ASD develop brains that are too big because inordinate growth may occur early. Studies document that such enlargement may cause social deficits to emerge as early as the end of an ASD child's first year (Hazlett et al. 2017). Data compiled from 148 children with a variety of ASD risk factors demonstrates that enlargement of the cortex's surface (sometimes called the cerebral cortex), observable through imaging and occurring from six to twelve months after birth, presages full inflation of the brain between the first and second year. In other words, brain imaging can predict the likelihood of social deficits, an ASD hallmark, as early as a child's sixth month. Such early detection should accelerate ASD's diagnosis and treatment. Early diagnosis and treatment provide the best opportunity to better people with ASD's quality of life short of curing the malady and so should be central to ASD science and medicine until a cure or cures emerge.

Early Intervention

The search for ASD's holy grail of early intervention absent a cure or cures has motivated and continues to precipitate an avalanche of research because, as is evident perhaps to the point of redundancy throughout this book and other literature, the sooner treatment starts the better are prospects for improving quality of life (Center for Parent Information and Resources 2017). Education and therapies are targeted to children under or at age two. This focus embraces more than just ASD to include children with any developmental delay or disability and to strengthen their families. Such education and therapies treat the entire child by aiming to improve physicality, cognition, communication, sociability, and self-care. Nationwide, the Individuals with Disabilities Education Act (IDEA) defines parental rights as they apply to school services for children with ASD and other disabilities.

Diverse approaches are needed to meet the array of ASD signs and symptoms. The Centers for Disease Control and Prevention (CDC) highlights treatments that teach concrete skills at the earliest opportunity, urging parents to seek speech therapy for their children before awaiting an ASD diagnosis (Centers for Disease Control and Prevention 2015). In addition to speech, other life skills include learning to walk and interact with peers and adults as soon as feasible (National Institutes for Health 2009). The Early Start Denver Model (ESDM) targets behavioral therapies to children with ASD as young as one year. Therapies occupy children as many as twenty hours per week while offering parents many community services. The therapies, seldom lasting beyond a year, increased the average child's intelligence quotient (IQ) by 15.4 points during the first year whereas the study's children who received less intensive and alternative therapies gained just 4.4 IQ points on average. During the second year, which was the last for the few who got that far, improvements in ESDM children broadened to include gains in communication, motor, and life skills. Even children with severe ASD benefited from EDSM, especially when parents modeled it at home.

FUTURE DIRECTIONS

Research

Two conflicting trends complicate future research predictions. On one hand, interest in ASD appears to be widespread and increasing over time. Many factors are at work, including sympathetic media presentations and characterizations of people with ASD. Moreover, as physicians diagnose ever greater numbers of ASD cases, pressure builds to do more to improve treatments, and treatments depend on the latest research to be at their best. Increasing talk about ASD echoes within parent and advocacy groups and in public debates about how best to confront what appears to be an ASD epidemic in the United States and many other parts of the globe.

Although these factors foreshadow increases in research tempo and money in every suitably equipped agency, private facility, laboratory, and university, government funding is emerging as the obstacle In 2017, President Donald Trump proposed reducing the budget of the National Institutes of Health (NIH) by nearly $6 billion and the National Science Foundation (NSF) by more than 10 percent (Achenbach and Sun 2017). If enacted these cuts will cascade throughout science and medicine because the NIH and NSF fund other research through grants; but with less money, the size and number of grants will decrease. Scientists and physicians will have no choice but to cancel many projects, including research that might have neared a breakthrough with more time and money.

Future research will likely continue to investigate diagnosis, treatment, genetics, neurology, and the environment while funds shrink. More research into ASD's causes, physiology, pharmacology, genetics, neurology, onset, severity, complicating factors, comorbidities, and talk therapies, among other approaches to lessen signs and symptoms, and for the application of findings to people from birth to old age with ASD, is needed (Damiano et al. 2014).

There is also the need, now and in the future, for research into ASD's genetic and environmental factors, family dynamics, job training practices, earliest effective treatments, and treatments and prospects that encompass minorities with ASD, understudied groups like the aged, and those who vary markedly on the spectrum. Under these conditions, one or even a few therapies cannot hope to work on all or even most people with ASD.

Treatment and Funding

Increasing recognition of ASD's signs and symptoms escalates the need for research into treatments with a focus on those that work at the earliest age, that target their approach to the circumstances of each sufferer, and that promise the greatest improvements over time. Such goals need research on treatments that help people with ASD from birth to death, while clinicians and hospitals need to deliver the best treatments consistently so that no patient falls through the cracks (Perrin et al. 2012). ASD care must improve from its current spottiness and inefficiency (Payne 2014). Better outcomes are not automatic but depend on adequate and increasing funding.

As more children with ASD grow into adulthood, research on adult treatment is also needed (Left Brain, Right Brain 2009). Research on early interventions is important because physicians can diagnose most ASD cases before a child is three years old. But a focus on earliness does not benefit adults because no tests exist to pinpoint ASD in them. Efforts to increase funding, splintered or unified, will surely intensify in the future.

Public Attitudes and Legal Issues

Support and resources are available at varying levels. In many urban areas, parents need only visit a local website for lists of available resources. But rural areas are another matter. In ideal circumstances, parents might consult a national ASD organization, a group motivated by religious or civic sentiments, or a research university. But poor knowledge, coupled with omnipresent fears, results in stigmas against people with ASD (Walton 2013). The remedies are openness and candor.

Crime demands detection and punishment, outcomes that only laws can guarantee. Accordingly, the future of laws that safeguard disabled people, including people with ASD, are central to civilization. For example, laws already on the books protect and extend the rights of caregivers in charge of people with ASD and other disabled people. Proposed laws seek to specify and guarantee the rights of guardians who care for people with ASD and other disabled persons. Such codifications should expand laws to protect them into the future (Parental-Rights.org n.d.).

These expansions are in, and will in the future include, schools for several reasons. First, the number of ASD diagnoses is increasing, thereby pressing schools to accommodate these students in a variety of settings, whether through special education or mainstreaming. Second, schools will likely increase the number and use of individualized education plans (IEPs). Third, such interventions begin, and will in the future likely continue to occur, soon so that children with ASD receive the earliest instruction. The earliness movement, known as early intervention (EI), will likely be relabeled early childhood special education (ECSE), a reshuffling that applies only to ASD students in special education. Fourth, special education will likely cede ground to the growing desire to insert ASD students into traditional classes, a process known as mainstreaming. Fifth, preschool is expanding its numbers and in the future will likely continue to grow as the site of early intervention.

Laws will likely also expand in the future to define more precisely the extent of medical coverage for children with ASD, as seen during the Medicaid expansion under President Barack Obama (Tirella 2014). The Achieving a Better Life Experience (ABLE) Act, signed by Obama in December 2014, expanded options by allowing guardians of children with ASD to establish tax exempt savings to pay medical expenses. Additionally, more private insurers are extending coverage to the families of people with ASD. This expansion requires laws to enlarge future protections of people with ASD, whether children, adolescents, or adults. Growing interest in and concern for these adults has been widely reported.

CONCLUSION

The varied nature of ASD research is evident in studies that examine possible causes, whether biological alone or in concert with the environment. Previous chapters focus on various faulty genes that contribute to understanding ASD's biological and environmental factors like vaccines; parenting; exposure to peers or bullies at school; drugs, including alcohol and tobacco; gestational issues, like an expectant mother's medical history; exposure to toxins, including pesticides and other synthetic chemicals; the type and pace of learning; the presence, absence, or delay in rewards for good behavior; tactics to defuse tantrums and other inappropriate actions; and other external stimuli. These attributes receive coverage in other chapters. Not all factors are true causes, as is evident from the vaccine controversy highlighted in chapter 9 and exposing as fraud the claim that an old but effective version of the measles, mumps, and rubella (MMR) vaccine causes a rare condition in children with ASD. Such a range of research proclivities and outcomes complicates predictions about ASD's future. Attempts at prediction extend beyond questions about the type and funding of research to be favored in the future to include public attitudes and legal protections. These predictions, like those involving research, are difficult to flesh out in any detail. Again, education and parenting come to the fore. This chapter concludes with an invitation to read the case studies, glossary, and resources in the following pages.

REFERENCES

Achenbach, Joel, and Lena H. Sun. 2017. "Trump Budget Seeks Huge Cuts to Science and Medical Research, Disease Prevention." *Washington Post*, May 23. https://www.washingtonpost.com/news/to-your-health/wp/2017/05/22/trump-budget-seeks-huge-cuts-to-disease-prevention-and-medical-research-departments.

Autism Speaks. 2011. "Autism Speaks Funds Creation of World's Largest Autism Genome Library," October 13. https://www.autismspeaks.org/science/science-news/autism-speaks-funds-creation-world%E2%80%99s-largest-autism-genome-library.

Belluck, Pam. 2014. "Study Finds That Brains with Autism Fail to Trim Synapses as They Develop." *New York Times*, August 21. https://www.nytimes.com/2014/08/22/health/brains-of-autistic-children-have-too-many-synapses-study-suggests.html.

Center for Parent Information and Resources. 2017. "Overview of Early Intervention," September 1. http://www.parentcenterhub.org/ei-overview/.

Centers for Disease Control and Prevention. 2015. "Autism Spectrum Disorder: Treatment." https://www.cdc.gov/ncbddd/autism/treatment .html.

Damiano, Cara R., Carla A. Mazefsky, Susan B. White, and Gabriel S. Dichter. 2014. "Future Directions for Autism Spectrum Disorders." *Journal of Clinical Child & Adolescent Psychology* 43, no. 5 (September–October): 828–843.

Hazlett, Heather Cody, H. Gu, B. C. Munsell, S. H. Kim, M. Styner, J. J. Wolff, J. T. Elison, et al. 2017. "Early Brain Development in Infants at High Risk for Autism Spectrum Disorder." *Nature* 542, no. 7641 (February 15): 348–351.

Left Brain, Right Brain. 2009. "Autism Research Funding: Who Is Paying and How Much?" July 21. https://leftbrainrightbrain.co.uk/2009/07/21 /autism-research-funding-who-is-paying-and-how-much/.

National Institutes for Health. 2009. "Autism Intervention for Toddlers Improves Developmental Outcomes." Science Update, December 8. https://www.nimh.nih.gov/archive/news/2009/autism-intervention -for-toddlers-improves-developmental-outcomes.shtml.

ParentalRights.org. n.d. "Rights for Parents with Disabilities." https:// parentalrights.org/disabilities/.

Payne, Tom. 2014. "Autism Care Standards Need to Be Improved, Says Nice." *The Guardian*, January 21. https://www.theguardian.com /society/2014/jan/21/autism-care-standards-need-to-be-improved -nice.

Perrin, James M., Daniel L. Coury, Nancy Jones, and Clara Lajonchere. 2012. "The Autism Treatment Network and Autism Intervention Research Network on Physical Health: Future Directions." *Pediatrics* 130, no. Supplement 2 (November).

Scripps Research Institute. 2015. "Mechanism for Altered Brain Pattern of Brain Growth in Autism Spectrum Disorder Discovered." Science Daily, July 15. https://www.sciencedaily.com/releases/2015/07 /150715155428.htm.

Scripps Research Institute. 2016. "Origin of Synaptic Pruning Process Linked to Learning, Autism and Schizophrenia Identified." Science Daily, May 2. https://www.sciencedaily.com/releases/2016/05 /160502161118.htm.

Tirella, Susan E. 2014. "Changes Made to Policy to Affect Thousands of Children with ASD." *Autism Parenting Magazine*, October. https:// www.autismparentingmagazine.com/policy-affect-thousands -children-asd/.

Walton, Lesa. 2013. "Changing Attitudes and Lives." *Learning Disabilities Today*. April 2. https://www.learningdisabilitytoday.co.uk/changing -attitudes-and-lives.

Case Illustrations

JOHN: CLASSIC SIGNS AND SYMPTOMS

Mary and her husband Ronald conceive a child, and after a normal gestation she gives birth to a son. The couple name him John after his paternal grandfather. The parents delight in nurturing him, and he begins to walk and talk around his first birthday. Within a few months, however, he begins to regress, especially in speech. He speaks seldom, even to his parents, refusing to acknowledge their questions. Both parents begin to suspect him of ignoring them. He rarely makes eye contact with anyone. His parents feel enormous distress because they have done everything to bond with him; yet now he is distancing himself from them.

Reluctant to tell anyone for fear of being branded substandard parents, Mary and Ronald first try to adjust to this new situation and to calm their nerves. Nonetheless, they come to conclude that John must see his pediatrician, Dr. Rachel Samuelson. At the office, they tell her of their fears and distress. Scrutinizing John to assess his minimal language, his refusal to make eye contact with her, his body language, and his general withdrawal, Dr. Samuelson concludes that he is developmentally delayed and counsel Mary and Ronald to take him to Dr. Richard Peterson, a specialist in a neighboring city.

After examining John, Dr. Peterson orders several tests, both physical and psychological. Physical tests include the measurement of John's head circumference in an attempt to detect either inordinate smallness (microcephaly) or largeness (macrocephaly). Both deviations from the norm may signal trouble. Too small a skull houses too small a brain, a condition linked to autism spectrum disorder (ASD). No better is macrocephaly, which sometimes results from the retention of too many synapses in the brain. This problem usually occurs in adolescence and is atypical at younger ages.

Nonetheless, caution dictates that Dr. Peterson dismiss no possibility too quickly.

Other physical tests are necessary. For example, a person with ASD usually has impaired coordination, balance, muscle tone (hypotonia), and muscle strength. These conditions, especially inadequate tone and strength, are evident early, allowing Dr. Peterson to test John for hypotonia, a potential cause of the other defects. Excessive clumsiness (dyspraxia) may derive from hypotonia, and Dr. Peterson tests John for it as well. More generally, autistic people, including those as young as John, may display an array of movement disorders such as tics, speech abnormalities, and overall poor coordination. Dr. Peterson measures all these movement deficits without instruments. Instead he watches and listens to John while interacting with him to spot these deficiencies. The specialist also asks Mary and Ronald whether they have witnessed these problems in John. Through observation and parental information, Dr. Peterson identifies Tourette's syndrome in John because his tics are too obvious for the doctor or Mary and John to ignore. Tourette's syndrome is a comorbid condition that overlaps with ASD. If John has seizures, he may suffer from epilepsy, another comorbidity, a possibility that Dr. Peterson rules out. Other physical signs and symptoms of ASD include insensitivity or hypersensitivity to touch. Dr. Peterson tests for all these particulars because ASD is, at its core, a neurological condition.

Physical measurements are not the lone tests because psychological assessments may also have value. Mary and Ronald are especially helpful here because they detail John's behavior verbally and in written tests that Dr. Peterson and other experts administer. Several written tests are on the market, including various attempts to quantify cognition. These tests derive from the intelligence quotient (IQ) tests invented in the United States early in the twentieth century. These derivatives include the Wechsler scale, the differential ability scale, the autism spectrum quotient, the adaptive behavior profile, various communication profiles, the childhood autism rating scale, the autism diagnostic interview, and the autism diagnostic observation schedule. Each has strengths and weaknesses that guide Dr. Peterson and colleagues in evaluating it. Data from these biological and psychological tests lead Dr. Peterson to diagnose John with ASD and to counsel his parents to coordinate treatments with his pediatrician and other doctors.

Analysis

This book, notably in Chapter 1's sections "Toward a Definition of Autism" and "ASD in Children and Adults" and in Chapter 4, notes ASD's early onset, a circumstance evident in this case study. John displays classic signs and symptoms, especially social deficits and language regression, described in Chapter 4's sections "Social Deficits as Signs and Symptoms" and "Language and Communication Deficits." Chapter 7's section "Family" emphasizes parents' role in detecting ASD signs and symptoms and in seeking medical attention, circumstances illustrated in this case study. Chapter 5's section "Diagnosis" describes several tests used to diagnose ASD, as this case study underscores.

John's parents respond prudently to their observations and concerns about their son by taking him to their pediatrician. She in turn observes John, realizing the need for a specialist to examine him. Only after a thorough consultation with the parents and observations of John does Dr. Peterson diagnose him with ASD. Dr. Peterson does not attempt to treat John alone. Rather he realizes the value of collaboration with other doctors. Accordingly this case study emphasizes not merely the parents' deliberate and careful actions, but those of John's doctors. Such an approach should give John the best opportunity for lessening his signs and symptoms, though the path toward treatment and management is lifelong because ASD does not have a cure.

HEATHER: EDUCATION AND EMPLOYMENT

As is common among adolescents, Heather, who has ASD, begins to formulate career objectives in high school. As career plans begin to crystallize, she approaches her guidance counselor, Mark Johnson, for advice. Like many counselors, he is a resource for information about careers and higher education. In this context, Heather wants his advice about colleges and universities. Mr. Johnson shifts in his chair at this request because he had not considered the possibility that Heather might aspire to a college degree. Nonetheless he helps her survey options, including the diversity of public and private colleges and universities in the United States, prospects for financial aid, school rankings, in-state versus out-of-state tuition for public institutions, and other factors. These options stimulate Heather to request information about graduate school in addition to undergraduate education because she hopes to become a librarian and knows that a master's degree is usually necessary for such positions. Mr. Johnson shifts gears accordingly despite his surprise to learn that Heather may not be content with merely a bachelor's degree. His unease stems partly from his conviction that graduate training may be too difficult for an individual with ASD.

Armed with information, Heather begins seeking admission to several universities with master's programs in library and information sciences, with the aim of pursuing undergraduate and graduate studies at the same institution. This hope leads her to favor the state land grant university because of its comprehensive undergraduate and graduate programs. Gaining admission, she earns a bachelor of arts degree in liberal studies and two years later a master's in library and information sciences (MLIS).

These degrees position Heather for a solid career because the university is the flagship institution in the state, is a source of regional pride, and has a stellar academic and athletic reputation. It is not among the elitist universities, but it is the best in the state and on par with excellent public universities throughout the United States. Given these strengths, Heather expects her hard work and ambitions to pay dividends. She applies for positions at several public libraries, reaping a handful of interviews. These interviews are not arduous, but Heather is unhappy that the prospective employers pigeonhole her as a cipher who will shelve books and perform other mundane tasks. She believes her education and achievements position her to be a reference librarian or another large cog in the machine. Interviewers sense her discomfort, and only one library offers her a job. Student debts compel her to accept even though the job entails little more than transferring calls to the reference desk and checking out books to patrons. Heather complies but within six months begins to apply elsewhere because her job appears to offer no prospects for promotion. The targeted libraries discard her application because she appears to be a job jumper, having held her current position only half a year. The path toward upward mobility blocked, Heather languishes at her job.

Analysis

Heather's situation mirrors that of many people with ASD who seek an education and employment. Chapter 6's section "Employment" details their problems. As an example of an autistic person, Heather might be thought atypical. For example, some 80 percent of autistic people are males, as noted in Chapter 1's section "ASD in Children and Adults," putting Heather in the minority. Moreover, as she begins thinking about career possibilities, Heather might be thought odd because she does not gravitate toward simple, repetitive jobs sometimes thought ideal for autistic people because of their preference for repetition and sameness, as noted in Chapter 6's section "Employment." Instead she considers careers that require collegiate training even though the majority of autistic people complete their education in high school. Moving beyond Heather's immediate circumstances, the tendency to end schooling at the end of grade 12 does not differentiate autistics from neurotypical individuals because college graduates, regardless of special considerations, are a minority of

America's population. More broadly, Heather bucks common perceptions of autistic people because she wants a career with the possibility of increasing responsibilities and concurrent gains in income whereas research, summarized in Chapter 6's section "Employment," indicates that most people with ASD are not motivated by money or aspirations for promotion and managerial authority. In fact, not all autistic people possess the skills to convince employers to hire them let alone the social savvy to manage subordinates. Again, some neurotypical individuals also lack these skills.

In other ways, however, Heather's story is typical of those with ASD. Her guidance counselor's surprise that she wants to pursue a college education typifies many people's assumptions about autistics' limitations. Such thinking is faulty, especially given the number of autistics who excel in their careers and sometimes have mathematical and technical proclivities. In fact, Mr. Johnson has no basis for such thoughts because Heather was not coasting through school but was taking challenging courses at every opportunity. Also too common is the perception of Heather's interviewers that she is suited for repetitive, simple tasks. Although such jobs satisfy some autistics, Heather's story makes clear that others hanker for challenges and responsibilities. Heather is also typical in facing not only a glass ceiling but concerns that she is not building a stable career but rather moving through a succession of jobs. A fragmented employment history, Chapter 6's section "Employment" emphasizes, typifies many autistics and contributes to their plight.

STEVE, LISA, JULIE, AND JENSEN: COPING WITH A FAMILY MEMBER WITH ASD

Lisa is the older sister of autistic brother Steve. Because of his later birth and disability, he is vulnerable to a greater degree than is Lisa. As parents, Julie and Jensen are attuned to differences in their children and worry more about Steve because of his youth and infirmity than might otherwise have been the case. Even though Lisa does her best to cater to Steve, she cannot help but grow jealous at the attention he receives. This jealousy requires an outlet so that she sometimes becomes quarrelsome. This misbehavior leads to excessive emotionalism and, coupled with Steve's ferocious tantrums, dismays Julie and Jensen almost beyond endurance. Their frayed nerves become raw so that their gentle dispositions sometimes falter. In frustration, Julie and Jensen sometimes bicker about mundane matters that ordinarily would not interest them.

These difficulties multiply as Jensen stays late at work even though his supervisor urges him to take time off to care for Steve. As an engineer, Jensen can adjust his schedule to meet family needs but instead chooses to linger at the office to delay his return home. Julie acknowledges the demands of her husband's job even though she knows that he can bend his schedule to the circumstances. She initially sympathizes with his comments that work is unusually busy, but over the next few months she comes to resent his absence as avoidance of his familial duties. She feels frustrated as family chores mount. Circumstances are worse because Julie also works outside the home, concretizing the problem of the double shift that plagues so many women who work to meet professional and family expectations. The load is especially heavy because Julie must work extra hours to bring home more money to help cover Steve's medical expenses.

Social deficits hinder Steve from understanding and sympathizing with his mother's difficulties, but Lisa, being older and aware of family dynamics, intuits her mother's plight. Lisa tries to compensate by doing more chores, but these demands on her time and energy only increase her resentment toward Steve even though she knows he deserves no blame for the family's skewed interactions.

As problems mount, Julie and Jensen seek counseling, not just to improve the marriage but to equalize as much as possible their treatment of Lisa and Steve. The therapist, Rick Stevenson, listens intently as both parents inundate him with information. Julie and Jensen have not brought their children to this first session because of their wish not to burden him with too many details. Even without the children, the session is intense and wide ranging. At its end, Mr. Stevenson urges Julie and Jensen to bring Lisa and Steve the next time to allow him a fuller understanding of the family.

Julie and Jensen comply, and Lisa and Steve brace for their first encounter with Mr. Stevenson. Despite her hesitance to join the conversation, Lisa admits how difficult the past months have been on everyone. Mr. Stevenson, studying her body language, understands how roughly these months have treated her in addition to everyone else, and by session's end both therapist and family members acknowledge the scope of the problems and agree that more extensive and intensive therapy is necessary. Even Steve appears to be aware that difficulties surround him so that everyone understands the urgency of redoubling efforts to repair the family.

Analysis

This case study concretizes many of the issues in Chapter 7, acknowledging that families are inherently complicated as a function of human complexity. Yet ASD has added intricacies to this family. The marriage suffers, a common problem noted in Chapter 7's subsection "Effects on Marriage." As is too often true, marital problems affect the children. Many of these problems harm Lisa, who must bear the burden of being old enough to understand the underlying dynamics and young enough to have trouble containing her jealousy and resentment. The sibling rivalry evident in the relationship between Lisa and Steve is a topic explored in Chapter 7's subsection "Effects on Siblings." Julie and Jensen add to the burden by doting on Steve. Favoritism destabilizes a family because the children, and often the parents as well, perceive unevenness in attention and nurturing. Julie and Jensen aim to treat their children uniformly, but Steve's ASD tilts energy and effort toward him because his parents and even Lisa understand that his difficulties require extra care and hands-on supervision. Parents and Lisa go out of their way to help Steve, but his need for constant care frays everyone's patience.

This study underscores the difficulties that beset families with an autistic member. Julie and Jensen strive to be the best parents, and their intentions appear to be honorable. Yet Jensen shirks his responsibilities by dallying at work. Julie cannot be faulted for feeling neglected, and the couple is proactive in seeking counseling to improve their marriage and parenting. Mr. Stevenson listens to both parents and, not content to hear their story alone, seeks confirmation and additional perspectives by inviting the children to the second session. Such comprehensive efforts give this family the opportunity to correct problems, though the path toward improvement will be arduous.

DAVID: DRUG SIDE EFFECTS

David, a young boy with ASD, has comorbidities depression and anxiety. The two are serious conditions, and the days have passed when insensitive people can reasonably claim that a depressed person need only "snap out of it" to recover. Accordingly, David's child psychiatrist has prescribed an assortment of antidepressants and antianxiety medicines. Such combinations lessen some of David's signs and symptoms but at costs to his health and psyche. Antidepressants and antianxiety medicines lead him to become obese.

David's attendance at Fairfield Elementary School only exacerbates his problems. His social deficits make him a target of bullies, whose taunting escalates as he gains weight. His social deficiencies prevent David from knowing how to evade or challenge these bullies. Teachers, counselors, and administrators, aware of his situation, intervene by chastising the bullies, but the tongue-lashing has little effect because of their pleasure in tormenting David. This intervention failing, Principal Sandra Evans calls his parents to share her concerns. The parents, expressing alarm, agree to meet her after school. Ms. Evans prepares for their arrival by asking David not to board the school bus so he may join the conference. Parents, David, and Ms. Evans gather in her office, where she recommends homeschooling to allow David to undergo more intensive interventions from his psychiatrist and therapist. She urges the parents to keep their son in school by enrolling him in online public education, a homeschooling alternative that preserves the content and standards that have defined his experiences at Fairfield. But the parents, products of public education, are ambivalent. Both had excelled in school in a variety of settings, whether in the classroom or in sports. They have long hoped that as David matures he might take an active role in school. Under these circumstances, the suggestion of homeschooling strikes them as a step backwards. Reluctantly they defer to Ms. Evans and enroll David in the state's virtual public schools. Free from bullying, he seems to adjust to the new experience, but his parents worry that online immersion is isolating him even more than had been the case at Fairfield. In this precarious position, his parents hope for success even as they feel powerless to reinsert him into the vigor and immediacy of in-person schooling.

Analysis

David's story amplifies Chapter 7's section "Family" by presenting his problems in the context of his parents' efforts to educate him in the least restrictive environment, a desire of many caregivers with special-needs children. This case study underscores the difficulties of such parents and children. On one hand, David's parents want him to develop socially, believing that school serves this purpose. On the other hand, they must protect David from bullies. This imperative leads them to homeschool David despite misgivings.

David's plight also illustrates that pharmacology is imperfect. As Chapter 5's subsection "Drug Therapies" makes clear, pharmaceuticals can enhance a physician's treatments for ASD. He or she does not target any medicine at ASD in the abstract but rather at signs and symptoms, which can be severe where comorbidities are present. Therapeutic drugs may reduce signs and symptoms, but they inevitably cause side effects. Some side effects are not alarming. For example, some medicines dry the mouth and tongue. The condition is unpleasant but does not endanger life. Rather it causes the sufferer to drink much water and to urinate often. No one would deem these problems inconsequential, but they are small.

Other side effects can be devastating. Among them is weight gain, a problem that has made David obese. Obesity can mar life at any age, but it seems particularly tragic in childhood because of its physical and psychological damage. David's obesity puts him at risk of several life-threatening conditions including heart disease, stroke, respiratory ailments, and some types of cancer, even though he is a child whose life should be long given the benefits of modern medicine. Beyond physical problems, David's psyche takes a beating from bullying. Even well adjusted children can crumble under such pressures, but David is especially vulnerable because his ASD has not given him the social skills to negate bullying. Under such pressures, homeschooling may be the best option for him.

PAUL: STRIVING FOR INDEPENDENCE

Thirty-year-old Paul has had three decades to develop mechanisms to minimize his ASD signs and symptoms. Minimization does not mean that Paul has few signs and symptoms, only that he has learned to mask them well enough that neurotypical people seldom suspect him of being atypical. Such masking requires enormous effort, which Paul summons every time he crosses paths with someone else.

A pizza store employee, he must interact with many people every day. Customers, coworkers, and managers invariably need his assistance. Occasionally he answers the phone and makes deliveries. These interactions regularly connect him with strangers. As with many autistics, these encounters challenge Paul, who must scrutinize strangers in hopes of detecting facial cues and other types of body language in attempting to understand them. That is, Paul spends much of his day trying to decode others' intentions so he can respond appropriately. Not every interaction requires strenuous attention and deliberation. The manager's signal to man the dishwasher sends Paul to it without hesitation so that no conscious decision is necessary. Other directives have the same effect so that Paul operates on autopilot part of the day. Such minimalism is impossible when he takes orders because some customers equivocate as they struggle to decide what to buy. They may place and then retract an order or ask Paul to recommend toppings or the pizza that will not cost too much money or satiate them too quickly while delivering the best nutrition. Such exchanges require him to think and respond quickly to requests, at least partly because any delay will increase the number of customers awaiting service.

Paul's courteous performance leads management to give him more responsibilities so that his workday is especially full. These evolving demands press Paul to double his efforts and drive toward the most prompt and efficient service. In keeping pace with these requirements, Paul earns a series of raises that allows him to afford an apartment in a middle-class neighborhood. This comfort, security, stability, and independence mark Paul as a hard worker on the ascent toward prosperity. Strangers who see him on an errand have no inkling of his ASD. His integration into the middle class concretizes the independence of many high functioning individuals with ASD.

Analysis

Like any disease, malady, condition, ailment, or affliction, ASD shapes lives. Particularly pertinent are living arrangements, a topic explored in Chapter 6's section "Employment." Because ASD is a spectrum, no single type of housing or number of people per dwelling can exhaust the possibilities. Nevertheless, living arrangements may be divided into two kinds. On one hand, autistics unable to care for themselves without assistance cannot live alone. This category includes children with ASD, no matter how gifted. Adults are a separate issue because they are not minors and may be able to make decisions without guidance. Nonetheless, adults who cannot meet the minimum standards of self-care cannot live alone. Independence is possible for others, autistic or neurotypical, as long as the money does not run out and laws are obeyed.

Paul is independent because he does his job well. In this sense, Paul is a counterweight to Heather, mentioned in the second case study. He illustrates that successful autistics adapt to their circumstances and learn new skills. In this respect, he reflects the traits necessary for anyone to succeed at work. Paul also contrasts to Heather because he does not crave her type of career. In this regard, he comes closer than Heather to the stereotype of the autistic worker as menial employee. Yet his story makes clear that such work does not limit him. He grows at his job, accepting more responsibilities as his supervisors gain confidence in him. In these ways, Paul is an example of the upward mobility to which people with ASD can aspire.

Glossary

Allele
One gene in a pair of genes.

Amygdala
The region of the brain that houses basic emotions like fear, aggression, and pleasure.

Antipsychotics
Drugs designed to minimize signs and symptoms of psychoses.

Aposteriori
Knowledge that derives from the senses.

Apriori
Knowledge that does not depend on the senses.

Autosome
Anon-sex chromosome.

Behavioral therapies
Talk therapies that aim to improve harmful behaviors associated with ASD or a mental health condition.

Biology
The natural science that studies life.

Biotechnology
The attempt to improve an organism by inserting a new gene or genes into it.

Brainstem
Portion of the brain that regulates the flow of chemicals between the brain and the rest of the body, thereby controlling breathing, heart rate, swallowing, blood pressure, consciousness, and sleepiness.

Central nervous system (CNS)
The totality of the body's nerves, including the brain. All vertebrates have a CNS of a brain and spinal cord.

Cerebellum
The region of the brain that coordinates the timing, sequence, and rate of muscle contractions.

Cesarean birth
The surgical delivery of a baby by cutting through the mother's abdomen in cases where baby, mother, or both are in danger.

Chromosome
A package of genes passed from parents to offspring as a means of distributing traits over time.

Circadian rhythm
A biological cycle that regulates sleep and wakefulness.

Comorbidity
The presence of two medical conditions in a patient.

Corpus callosum
The region of the brain that connects both halves (hemispheres) of the brain in a network of fibers (nerves) that shuttles electrochemical signals between hemispheres.

Cortex
The outermost region of the brain that gives humans consciousness.

Cortisol
A (nonanabolic) steroid hormone that regulates wakefulness by producing a surge in energy, typically during the morning to ready the body for the day's activities.

Cytoplasm
The entire cell in an organism minus the nucleus.

Deoxyribonucleic acid (DNA)
The macromolecule of heredity. It is a large sugar molecule composed of nucleotide bases.

Diagnosis
A process whereby a physician or other medical practitioner attempts to determine what is wrong with a patient.

Dominance
The expression of a gene in a pair of genes (alleles) whenever that gene is present in the pair.

Dyspraxia
A medical condition whereby a person has difficulty coordinating the muscles, causing clumsiness.

Empiricism
The conjecture that humans derive all knowledge through the senses.

Endocrine gland
A gland that releases a hormone or hormones into the blood for transit to other parts of the body.

Gastrointestinal system
Body system that comprises the buccal cavity, the pharynx, the esophagus, the stomach, and the duodenum, all of which cooperate to digest food.

Gene
A sequence of nucleotide bases that codes for production of a protein. Genes direct proteins to assemble every structure in an organism.

Gene therapy
The attempt to improve an organism through enhancement of favorable genes, silencing of harmful ones, or both. It is not now possible.

Genetics
The branch of biology that studies heredity.

Genome
The aggregate of all genes in an organism or the aggregate of all genes in a species. The second meaning is more widespread today.

Genotype
The aggregate of all genes in an organism. This meaning overlaps with the first definition of genome.

Gland
A bodily structure or organ that produces a hormone or hormones that regulate some part of the body.

Gluten
A complex of proteins found in the grains wheat, rye, barley, and triticale. Some people cannot properly digest gluten.

Hormone
A chemical produced by a gland to regulate activity in a group of cells.

Hypothalamus
A region of the brain that regulates the pituitary gland through production of hormones.

Hypotonia
Muscle weakness caused by inadequate muscle tone.

Immune system
A group of cells, tissues, and organs that patrols the body to guard against infection.

Intelligence quotient (IQ)
An attempt to quantify intelligence by putting a person's mental age in the numerator of a fraction and the chronological age in the denominator.

Macrocephaly
An abnormal enlargement of the brain, a condition in some people with ASD.

Microcephaly
An abnormal reduction in brain size, a condition in some people with ASD.

Monogenetic trait
A trait that depends on the expression of one gene.

Musculoskeletal system
The muscles, bones, and tissues that connect the two.

Mutation
A chemical change, usually harmful, to a gene.

Neuroendocrine system
A bodily system that includes the pineal gland, the pituitary gland, the pancreas, the ovaries in women or the testes in men, the thyroid gland, the parathyroid gland, the hypothalamus, and the adrenal glands.

Neurology
The study of nerves and their activity in the CNS.

Neuron
A cell that carries electrochemical signals (messages) from the brain to other parts of the body.

Neurosis
A mental condition in which anxiety limits the ability to cope with life's demands.

Neurotransmitter
A substance that carries an electrochemical signal across a synapse in the form of another chemical.

Nicotine
A toxin in tobacco that stimulates the body in small doses but causes many ailments, including some cancers and heart disease.

Nucleotide base
A molecule and component of DNA and RNA. The bases in DNA are guanine, thymine, cytosine, and adenine. The bases in RNA are the same except that uracil replaces thymine.

Nucleus
The center of a cell that may be thought of as the headquarters because it contains most of the genetic information to direct the cell.

Oxytocin
A hormone and neurotransmitter produced by the pituitary gland. Oxytocin shapes sociability and sexual behaviors. It stimulates contractions in a pregnant woman and milk production in her breasts.

Pesticide
A synthetic chemical designed to kill insects and animals, deemed harmful to humans or an aspect of economic production.

Phenotype
The aggregate of all physical traits in an organism.

Pineal gland
A structure in the brain that regulates sleep through production of the hormone melatonin.

Pituitary gland
A brain structure located at the base of the brain that regulates the body's growth and controls other endocrine glands through the production of several hormones.

Polygenetic trait
A trait that depends on the expression of more than one gene.

Pons
A network of nerves that connects upper and lower parts of the brain.

Prognosis
An attempt to predict the future course of a medical condition.

Psychosis
A mental condition that impairs a person's ability to distinguish reality from fantasy.

Rapid eye movement (REM)
The period during sleep when people dream.

Recessiveness
The expression of a gene in a pair of genes (alleles) only when that gene occupies both loci in the pair.

Refrigerator mom thesis
The now discredited hypothesis that cold, distant parents, especially mothers, cause ASD in their children.

Ribose nucleic acid (RNA)
Molecules that carry the instructions in DNA outside a cell's nucleus to direct protein synthesis in the cytoplasm.

Schizophrenia
A psychosis that usually appears in adolescence or young adulthood and may resemble ASD in presenting social deficits, language impairment, and poor eye contact with others.

Selective serotonin reuptake inhibitors (SSRIs)
Drugs that impair the brain's ability to reabsorb (reuptake) serotonin.

Serotonin
The neurotransmitter and hormone 5-hydroxyltryptamine that regulates the transmission of electrochemical signals between neurons, sets a person's mood, regulates the movement and elimination of wastes, causes nausea when a person ingests a toxin, causes osteoporosis when in excess, regulates the libido, and helps form blood clots.

Sign
A behavior that a physician might notice in a patient in attempting to diagnose a condition.

Stigma
A negative judgment formed about a person because of some attribute or behavior deemed inappropriate.

Symptom
A behavior that a patient might notice without the aid of a physician and that might lead a patient to consult a physician.

Synapse
A gap (junction) over which electrochemical signals move as they travel from the brain to other parts of the body.

Tantrum
An uncontrolled outpouring of rage usually confined to childhood.

Vaccination
The administration of a vaccine, a substance that causes the body to produce antibodies against a pathogen (germ) as a way of protecting a person from the disease caused by that pathogen.

Directory of Resources

BOOKS

Aitken, Kenneth J. 2018. *Evidence-Based Assessment in ASD (Autism Spectrum Disorder): What Is Available, What Is Appropriate and What Is 'Fit-for-Purpose.'* London and Philadelphia: Jessica Kingsley Publishers.

Booth, Janine. 2016. *Autism Equality in the Workplace: Removing Barriers and Challenging Discrimination.* London and Philadelphia: Jessica Kingsley Publishers.

Correa, Bernardo Barahona, and Rutger-Jan van der Gaag, eds. 2017. *Autism Spectrum Disorders in Adults.* Cham, Switzerland: Springer International.

Donvan, John, and Caren Zucker. 2016. *In a Different Key: The Story of Autism.* New York: Crown Publishers.

Feinstein, Adam. 2010. *A History of Autism: Conversations with the Pioneers.* West Sussex, UK: Wiley-Blackwell.

Grandin, Temple. 2003. *Autism: A Personal Perspective.* New York: Dekker.

Grandin, Temple, and Kate Duffy. 2008. *Developing Talents: Careers for Individuals with Asperger Syndrome and High-Functioning Autism.* Shawnee Mission, KS: Autism Asperger Publishing.

Grandin, Temple, and Richard Panek. 2014. *The Autistic Brain: Helping Different Kinds of Minds Succeed.* Boston: Houghton Mifflin Harcourt.

Hollander, Eric, Alexander Kolevzon, and Joseph T. Coyle. 2011. *Textbook of Autism Spectrum Disorders.* Washington, DC: American Psychiatric Publishing.

Hoopmann, Kathy. 2015. *The Essential Manual for Asperger Syndrome (ASD) in the Classroom: What Every Teacher Needs to Know.* London and Philadelphia: Jessica Kingsley Publishers.

Kaufman, Raun Kahlil. 2014. *Autism Breakthrough: The Groundbreaking Method That Has Helped Families All over the World.* New York: St. Martin's Press.

Leach, Debra. 2018. *Behavior Support for Students with ASD: Practical Help for 10 Common Challenges.* Baltimore: Paul H. Brookes Publishing.

Luiselli, James K., ed. 2014. *Children and Youth with Autism Spectrum Disorder (ASD): Recent Advances and Innovations in Assessment, Education, and Intervention.* New York: Oxford University Press.

Murray, Stuart. 2012. *Autism.* New York: Routledge.

Notbohm, Ellen. 2012. *Ten Things Every Child with Autism Wishes You Knew.* Arlington, TX: Future Horizons.

Perry, Nancy. 2009. *Adults on the Autism Spectrum Leave the Nest: Achieving Supported Independence.* London and Philadelphia: Jessica Kingsley Publishers.

Prizant, Barry M. 2016. *Uniquely Human: A Different Way of Seeing Autism.* London: Souvenir Press.

Rotatori, Anthony F., Festus E. Obiakor, and Sandra Burkhardt, eds. 2008. *Autism and Developmental Disabilities: Current Practices and Issues.* Bingley, UK: Emerald JAI.

Senator, Susan. 2016. *Autism Adulthood: Strategies and Insights for a Fulfilling Life.* New York: Skyhorse Publishing.

Shannon, Joyce Brennfleck, ed. 2011. *Autism and Pervasive Developmental Disorders Sourcebook.* 2nd ed. Detroit: Omnigraphics.

Shapiro, Bruce K., and Pasquale J. Accardo. 2008. *Autism Frontiers: Clinical Issues and Innovations.* Baltimore: Paul H. Brookes Publishing.

Silberman, Steve. 2016. *NeuroTribes: The Legacy of Autism and the Future of Neurodiversity.* New York: Avery.

Wexler, Alice. 2016. *Autism in a Decentered World.* New York: Routledge.

ARTICLES

Davis, Kim. 2004. "What's in a Name: Our Only Label Should Be Our Name: Avoiding Stereotypes." *The Reporter* 9, no. 2: 10–12, 24.

Grandin, Temple. 2000. "My Mind Is a Web Browser: How People with Autism Think." *Cerebrum* 2, no. 1 (Winter): 14–22.

Kester, Karen R., and Joseph M. Lucyshyn. 2018. "Cognitive Behavior Therapy to Treat Anxiety among Children with Autism Spectrum Disorders: A Systematic Review." *Research in Autism Spectrum Disorders* 52 (August): 37–50.

Phillips, K. L., L. A. Schieve, S. Visser, S. Boulet, A. J. Sharma, M. D. Kogan, C. A. Boyle, and M. Yeargin-Allsopp. 2014. "Prevalence and Impact of Unhealthy Weight in a National Sample of U.S. Adolescents with Autism and Other Learning and Behavioral Disabilities." *Maternal and Child Health Journal* 18, no. 8 (October): 1964–1975.

Sun, Xiang, and Carrie Allison. 2010. "A Review of Autism Spectrum Disorder in Asia." *Research in Autism Spectrum Disorders* 4, no. 2 (April–June): 156–167.

WEBSITES

"Autism Risk Higher in People with Gene Variant." 2008. National Institutes of Health, January 10. Accessed June 7, 2018. http://www.nih.gov/news-events/news-releases/autism-risk-higher-people-gene-variant.

"Autism Spectrum Disorder." 2015. National Institute of Mental Health, September. Accessed June 7, 2018. http://www.nimh.nih.gov/health/publications/autism-spectrum-disorder/index.shtml.

"Autism Spectrum Disorder (ASD)." 2018. Centers for Disease Control and Prevention, May 3. Accessed June 7, 2018. http://www.cdc.gov/ncbddd/autism/index.html.

Bakare, Muideen O. 2014. "Current Situation of Autism Spectrum Disorders (ASD) in Africa—A Review." Accessed August 25, 2017. http://grand.tghn.org/site_media/media/medialibrary/2014/12/bakare_autism_spectrum_disorders_in_Africa.pdf.

Barna, Mark. 2017. "Everything Worth Knowing about … Autism Spectrum Disorder." *Discover*, June 19. Accessed June 7, 2018. http://discovermagazine.com/2017/jul-aug/autism-spectrum-disorder.

Barna, Mark. 2018. "Spotting Autism Sooner." *Discover*, January/February. Accessed June 7, 2018. http://discovermagazine.com/2018/janfeb/61-spotting-autism-sooner.

Boyse, Kayla. 2008. "Autism, Autism Spectrum Disorders (ASD) and Pervasive Developmental Disorders (PDD)." Michigan Medicine, University of Michigan, December. Accessed June 7, 2018. http://www.med.umich.edu/yourchild/topics/autism.htm.

Donvan, John, and Caren Zucker. 2010. "Autism's First Child." *The Atlantic*, October. Accessed June 7, 2018. http://www.theatlantic.com/magazine/archive/2010/10/autisms-first-child/308227.

Engelking, Carl. 2014. "Genetics May Explain Why Autism Is More Common in Boys." *Discover*, February 27. Accessed August 25, 2017. http://blogs.discovermagazine.com/d-brief/2014/02/27/genetics-may-explain-why-autism-is-more-common-in-boys/#.WZ78Ztqrjkg.

Hadhazy, Adam. 2011. "Unmasking Autism." *Discover*, Fall. Accessed June 7, 2018. http://discovermagazine.com/2011/brain/unmasking-autism.

McGovern, Cammie. 2017. "Looking into the Future for a Child with Autism." *New York Times*, August 31. Accessed June 7, 2018. http://www.nytimes.com/2017/08/31/well/family/looking-into-the-future-for-a-child-with-autism.html.

Mooney, Chris. 2009. "Why Does the Vaccine/Autism Controversy Live On?" *Discover*, May 6. Accessed June 7, 2018. http://discovermagazine.com/2009/jun/06/why-does-vaccine-autism-controversy-live-on.

National Institute of Mental Health. n.d. "Autism Spectrum Disorder." Accessed August 25, 2017. http://www.nimh.nih.gov/health/topics/autism-spectrum-disorders-asd/index.shtml.

Neimark, Jill. 2007. "Autism: It's Not Just in the Head." *Discover*, March 22. Accessed June 7, 2018. http://discovermagazine.com/2007/apr/autism-it2019s-not-just-in-the-head.

Pratt, Cathy. 2017. "Characteristics of Individuals with an Autism Spectrum Disorder (ASD)." *The Reporter*. Accessed June 7, 2018. http://iidc.indiana.edu/pages/characteristics.

Pratt, Cathy. 2018. "Autism Awareness Month: Tips for Working with Individuals on the Autism Spectrum." *IRCA Reporter E-Newsletter*. Accessed June 7, 2018. http://www.iidc.indiana.edu/pages/autism-awareness-month-a-facts-andtips-for-working-with-individuals-on-the-autism-spectrum.

Robinson, John Elder. 2018. "Is the Definition of Autism Too Broad?" *Psychology Today*, June 2. Accessed June 7, 2018. http://www.psychologytoday.com/us/blog/my-life-aspergers/201806/is-the-definition-autism-too-broad.

Shapin, Steven. 2016. "Seeing the Spectrum: A New History of Autism." *New Yorker*, January 25. Accessed June 7, 2018. http://www.newyorker.com/magazine/2016/01/25/seeing-the-spectrum.

Siegel, Bryna. 2018. "What Autism Isn't." *Psychology Today*, May 30. Accessed June 7, 2018. http://www.psychologytoday.com/us/blog/the-politics-autism/201805/what-autism-isnt.

Stuart-Hamilton, Ian. 2013. "People with Autism Spectrum Disorder Take Things Literally." *Psychology Today*, April 7. Accessed June 7, 2018. http://www.psychologytoday.com/us/blog/the-gift-aging/201304/people-autism-spectrum-disorder-take-things-literally.

Szalawitz, Maia. 2016. "Autism—It's Different in Girls." *Scientific American*, March 1. Accessed June 7, 2018. http://www.scientificamerican.com/article/autism-it-s-different-in-girls.

Willingham, Emily. 2012. "Is Autism an 'Epidemic' or Are We Just Noticing More People Who Have It?" *Discover*, July 11. Accessed June 7, 2018. http://blogs.discovermagazine.com/crux/2012/07/11/is-autism-an-epidemic-or-are-we-just-noticing-more-people-who-have-it/#.wxles9qrjkg.

Zimmer, Carl. 2012. "The Brain: The Troublesome Bloom of Autism." *Discover*, March 5. Accessed June 7, 2018. http://discovermagazine.com/2012/mar.07-the-brain-troublesome-bloom-autism.

ORGANIZATIONS

American Psychiatric Association: http://www.psychiatry.org.
Association for Science in Autism Treatment: http://www.asatonline.org.
Autism-Europe: http://www.autismeurope.org.
Autism National Committee: http://www.autcom.org.
Autism Network International: http://autismnetworkinternational.org.
Autism Research Institute: http://www.autism.com.
Autism Resource Centre: http://www.autism.org.sg.
Autism Society: http://www.autism-society.org.
Autism Speaks: http://www.autismspeaks.org.
Autistic Self Advocacy Network: http://autisticadvocacy.org.
Center for Autism and Related Disorders: http://www.centerforautism.com.
Centers for Disease Control and Prevention: http://www.cdc.gov.
Families for Early Autism Treatment: http://www.feat.org.
National Autism Association: http://nationalautismassociation.org.
National Autistic Society: http://www.autism.org.uk.
National Institute of Mental Health: http://www.nimh.nih.gov.
Organization for Autism Research: http://www.researchautism.org.
Parents of Autistic Children Autism Services: http://www.poac.net.
Talk about Curing Autism: http://tacanow.org.
World Autism Organisation: http://worldautismorganisation.com.
World Health Organization: http://www.who.int.

Index

About the Author

Christopher M. Cumo, PhD, is a historian with interests in science and medicine. His previous books with ABC-CLIO include *Science and Technology in 20th-Century American Life* (2007), *Foods That Changed History: How Foods Shaped Civilization from the Ancient World to the Present* (2015), and *The Ongoing Columbian Exchange: Stories of Biological and Economic Transfer in World History* (2015). He also edited the *Encyclopedia of Cultivated Plants: From Acacia to Zinnia* (2013).